MEAL PREP COOKBOOK

Quick and Easy Ketogenic Recipes You Can Prep Ahead to Save Time

(30 + Delicious Easy Recipes for the Whole Family)

Juanita Jenkins

Published by Alex Howard

© **Juanita Jenkins**

All Rights Reserved

Meal Prep Cookbook: Quick and Easy Ketogenic Recipes You Can Prep Ahead to Save Time (30 + Delicious Easy Recipes for the Whole Family)

ISBN 978-1-990169-68-7

All rights reserved. No part of this guide may be reproduced in any form without permission in writing from the publisher except in the case of brief quotations embodied in critical articles or reviews.

Legal & Disclaimer

The information contained in this book is not designed to replace or take the place of any form of medicine or professional medical advice. The information in this book has been provided for educational and entertainment purposes only.

The information contained in this book has been compiled from sources deemed reliable, and it is accurate to the best of the Author's knowledge; however, the Author cannot guarantee its accuracy and validity and cannot be held liable for any errors or omissions. Changes are periodically made to this book. You must consult your doctor or get professional medical advice before using any of the suggested remedies, techniques, or information in this book.

Table of contents

Part 1 1
Introduction 2
A quick overview of the Ketogenic Diet 3
Why a new energy source is crucial for a healthy body 6
The health benefits of the Ketogenic Diet 8
Which foods should and should not be eaten on the Ketogenic Diet? 9
The best ways to cook food on the Ketogenic Diet 14
DAY-1 BREAKFAST 15
Delicious Mexican Frittata 15
DAY-1 LUNCH 17
Tasty Chicken Guacamole Salad 17
DAY-1 DINNER 19
Flavorful Chicken Piccata 19
DAY-2 BREAKFAST 20
Healthy Egg Breakfast Muffins 20
DAY-2 LUNCH 23
Creamy Cheesy Cauliflower Mash 23
DAY-2 DINNER 25
Cauliflower Cheese Casserole 25
DAY-3 BREAKFAST 26
Jalapeno Muffins 26

DAY-3 LUNCH 29

Bacon Avocado Chicken Salad 29

DAY-3 DINNER 31

Perfect Bacon Chicken 31

DAY-4 BREAKFAST 32

Easy Breakfast Bowl 32

DAY-4 LUNCH 34

Creamy Egg Salad 34

DAY-4 DINNER 36

Quick Cherry Tomato Frittata 36

DAY-5 BREAKFAST 37

Egg Breakfast Casserole 37

DAY-5 LUNCH 39

Chicken Basil Salad 39

DAY-5DINNER 40

Smoked Paprika Chicken 40

DAY-6 BREAKFAST 41

Almond Blueberry Muffins 41

DAY-6 LUNCH 42

Mayo Shrimp Cilantro Salad 42

DAY-6 DINNER 44

Simple Coconut Shrimp 44

DAY-7 BREAKFAST 45

Cheddar Broccoli Bread 45
DAY-7 LUNCH 46
Flavorful Tuna Salad 46
DAY-7 DINNER 48
Tuna Egg Bake 48
DAY-8 BREAKFAST 49
Delicious Ricotta Omelet 49
DAY-8 LUNCH 51
Flavorful Citrusy Shrimp 51
DAY-8 DINNER 53
Simple Old Bay Seasoned Shrimp 53
DAY-9 BREAKFAST 54
Olive Bacon Quiche 54
DAY-9 LUNCH 56
Easy Cabbage Noodles 56
DAY-9 DINNER 57
Cauliflower Cheese Casserole 57
DAY-10 BREAKFAST 59
Coconut Waffles 59
DAY-10 LUNCH 61
Curried Chicken Salad 61
DAY-10 DINNER 63
Cheese Broccoli Soup 63

DAY-11 BREAKFAST 64
Easy Egg Loaf 64
DAY-11 LUNCH 66
Almond Chicken Salad 66
DAY-11 DINNER 67
Shrimp Mushroom Soup 67
DAY-12 BREAKFAST 68
Delicious Breakfast Cookies 68
DAY-12 LUNCH 70
Cucumber Tuna Salad 70
DAY-12 DINNER 71
Delicious Ranch Chicken 71
DAY-13 BREAKFAST 72
Bacon Cheese Bread 72
DAY-13 LUNCH 74
Chili Garlic Shrimp 74
DAY-13 DINNER 75
Pesto Cheese Salmon 75
DAY-14 BREAKFAST 76
Coconut Chia Pudding 76
DAY-14 LUNCH 78
Avocado Bacon Soup 78
DAY-14 DINNER 80

Lemon Parmesan Salmon	80
DAY-15 BREAKFAST	81
Spinach Bacon Frittata	81
DAY-15 LUNCH	83
Italian Pepperoni Avocado Salad	83
DAY-15 DINNER	84
Garlic Onion Pork Tenderloin	84
DAY-16 BREAKFAST	85
Healthy Coconut Porridge	85
DAY-16 LUNCH	87
Cilantro Shrimp Avocado Salad	87
DAY-16 DINNER	89
Lemon Garlic Chicken	89
DAY-17 BREAKFAST	90
Bacon Avocado Quiche	90
DAY-17 LUNCH	92
Perfect Geek Salad	92
DAY-17 DINNER	93
Zucchini Cheese Casserole	93
DAY-18 BREAKFAST	94
Healthy Spinach Quiche	94
DAY-18 LUNCH	95
Healthy Mediterranean Salad	95

DAY-18 DINNER 97
Tasty Pumpkin Spiced Soup 97
DAY-19 BREAKFAST 98
Almond Pumpkin Pancake 98
DAY-19 LUNCH 100
Refreshing Creamy Cucumber Salad 100
DAY-19 DINNER 101
Herb Chicken 101
DAY-20 BREAKFAST 102
Blueberry Almond Coconut Flour Casserole 102
DAY-20 LUNCH 104
Delicious Zucchini Soup 104
DAY-20 DINNER 106
Zucchini Cheese Gratin 106
DAY-21 BREAKFAST 107
Creamy Egg Scrambled 107
DAY-21 LUNCH 109
Easy Chicken Fajitas 109
DAY-21 DINNER 111
Zucchini Noodles 111
DAY-22 BREAKFAST 112
Cauliflower Cheese Bread 112
DAY-22 LUNCH 114

Mayo Cabbage Coleslaw	114
DAY-22 DINNER	116
Cauliflower Cheese Gratin	116
DAY-23 BREAKFAST	117
Herb Cauliflower Bread	117
DAY-23 LUNCH	119
Cabbage Dill Cucumber Salad	119
DAY-23 DINNER	121
Cheese Cauliflower Rice	121
DAY-24 BREAKFAST	122
Vanilla protein Muffins	122
DAY-24 LUNCH	124
Healthy Coconut Spinach Soup	124
DAY-24 DINNER	126
Baked Broccoli	126
DAY-25 BREAKFAST	127
Coconut Kale Muffins	127
DAY-25 LUNCH	129
Garlic Herb Baked Mushrooms	129
DAY-25 DINNER	131
Parmesan Spinach Pie	131
DAY-26 BREAKFAST	132
Spicy & Creamy Egg Scrambled	132

DAY-26 LUNCH	134
Creamy Cauliflower Broccoli Mashed	134
DAY-26 DINNER	135
Almond Jalapeno Pizza	135
DAY-27 BREAKFAST	136
Cinnamon Cream Egg Scrambled	136
DAY-27 LUNCH	137
Paprika Egg Cucumber Salad	137
DAY-27 DINNER	139
Spinach Casserole	139
DAY-28 BREAKFAST	140
Flavorful Cheese Quiche	140
DAY-28 LUNCH	142
Easy Caesar Salad	142
DAY-28 DINNER	143
Cheese Chicken Casserole	143
DAY-29 BREAKFAST	144
Tasty Cauliflower Frittata	144
DAY-29 LUNCH	146
Flavors Squash Soup	146
DAY-29 DINNER	147
Spicy Chicken Curry	147
DAY-30 BREAKFAST	148

Mushroom Asparagus Frittata 148

DAY-30 LUNCH 150

Simple Broccoli Omelet... 150

DAY-30 DINNER... 152

Meatloaf 152

Part 2 154

Introduction 155

CHAPTER ONE 160

CHAPTER TWO: Eating Clean.................................. 167

CHAPTER THREE 174

Breakfast... 174

Oatmeal with veggie, coconut and maple sautéed apples (gluten-free and vegan) 177

Healthy banana bread breakfast cookies 179

Stuffed zucchinis with taco filling............................ 180

Berry, arugula and quinoa salad with lemon-chia seed dressing 184

Soba noodles with kale, silvered Brussels sprouts and sesame dressing...............**Error! Bookmark not defined.**

Black bean plantain veggie burgers with onion and chipotle spice ....**Error! Bookmark not defined.**

Part 1

Introduction

The Ketogenic Diet is not a new way of eating in the world, but it is certainly a style of eating that has rightfully attracted a lot of attention from people who knew very little about it before. Considering how busy our current lifestyles are at the moment, it is understandable that people are finding it very difficult to match eating, fitness, stress-balance, and their family lives in a perfect mix. In fact, it is almost impossible to create an atmosphere where all of these things come together in the perfect way. Because so many people have such a difficult time prepping their everyday lives, one of the first things that goes out the window when it comes to balance is food.

The kind of food that we eat in the modern world revolves around things that are super quick to make, full of intense flavors, such as salt and sugar, and also full of additive and preservatives, so that they can last us a long time and we won't have to go grocery shopping often. Although it is certainly understandable that people are doing everything they can to balance their lives with their budget, when we ruin the way that we eat and the way that we nourish our bodies, we essential ruin the most important thing on a daily basis.

A body that has not been treated properly will lack energy, cause anxiety and depression, and it will also not be able to focus for long periods of time, which mean that our work lives will also have to suffer as a result.

This is not good, and in the long run, could be the cause of higher levels of anxiety in people and a loss of hope for a healthier life with less weight. However, the Ketogenic Diet is a way of eating that can truly help people overcome their poor eating habits, and could also show them a new style of living where individuals can form their own eating schedules, while still sticking to a diet that is easy to manage and easy to prepare.

A QUICK OVERVIEW OF THE KETOGENIC DIET

Before we move on to discuss how you can prepare for the Ketogenic Diet, we must first discuss what this diet actually is, what makes it so special, and which parts of this way of eating are the most crucial ones when it comes to living a healthier lifestyle. The diet itself is, luckily, not difficult to understand, but the more you know about it, the easier it will be for you to adapt and to get the most out of this style of eating.

The Ketogenic Diet is a diet that is comprised of wholefoods and high fat. It first appeared as a diet that was found to be able to help children with epilepsy problems, and was then extended to the wider public because there were a number of other health benefits that were discovered along the way. For the wider public, it is the chemistry behind the diet that makes it so useful for the wider masses, and why it is so effective when it comes to weight loss.

The chemistry behind this diet has to do with carbohydrates and energy sources of our bodies, which not only dictate our actual energy levels, but they are also dictate our weight, mood, and other health issues. Namely, it is often well-known to people that carbohydrates are our main source of energy. Whenever your body needs energy to do anything, it will always go to your carbohydrate sources first, and will use them all up entirely before it even tries to move on to another energy source. The reason why the body really loves carbs as energy is because carbs are super easy to break down and the use. It is very little effort from your body to select a group of carbs and create a burst of energy. Carbs are not bad for you though! Every aspect of food has its own positive and negative takes on the human body, but the thing that is important is to stick to the sources that are healthies and that will bring your body the best results.

However, there is a problem when it comes to carbohydrates. The problem is that we usually takes these carbs from food sources that are really not healthy for our bodies at all. This is usually through fast food, drinks, and desserts. Ever notice that it is precisely these foods that we so often crave? Some of the reasons for this are because our brain craves an instant source of happiness to make us happier faster, but the other side of the truth is precisely the source of energy that comes from carbohydrates. However, the other problem is the fact that our usual day jobs are almost always sedentary. We don't move nearly as much as people used to move before, which means that we are actually gaining weight much faster than previous generations. This is obviously very bad for our health, which is why we need to make a change in our life that will not ruin the health of our bodies.

The way to deal with this is with the help of the Ketogenic Diet. This diet is based on entirely wholefoods, especially those that are in season, and it is also based on the kind of diet that is truly high in fats. The reason why this is such good news for your body is because wholefoods are all we have left to make sure that we are feeding our bodies with the nutrients and the minerals that will actually be able to make us healthier overall. The great thing about the Ketogenic Diet is that the wholefoods that you choose to make your food from are always encouraged to be those that are in season. This is great for a number of reasons. One of those reasons is the fact that foods that are in season are cheaper than those that are imported from far places around the world, and which obviously cost more to arrive to their destination. This is also not good because these foods often have dangerous preservatives in order to make them last longer, but which in turn have negative effects on our bodies. Also, it is much easier to prepare your meals with wholefoods that are easy for you to purchase, and especially those that you can purchase from your local wholefoods producers, which also ensures that you are helping smaller agricultural businesses to succeed. Therefore, there are many positive reasons why the Ketogenic Diet is great both for the individual and for their environment.

WHY A NEW ENERGY SOURCE IS CRUCIAL FOR A HEALTHY BODY

Our bodies really love to stay in a situation that is super predictable. This is because our bodies don't like to be caught in surprise, because this means that the body needs to find a new way to manage itself and to deal with the environment. Whenever something new happens, our body is certainly great at adapting to the new situation, but it is safe to say that it is definitely not something that it wants to do. However, the thing that few people are aware of is that our body has a number of energy sources that it can use to make sure that everything is constantly in order. We already mentioned that carbs are the body's favorite source of energy, but the second favorite source of energy that our body can use is our own fat. However, the body will not try to use any of the fat storages that we have until it has completely used up all of the available carbs. This is because carbs are both easy to store and easy to burn, and also because we rarely reach a point in our lives where we will naturally use up all of the carbs inside of our system and finally make our body shift to using fat. This is because of the problem of modern day life that we have previously mentioned, where we live lives where we don't really use up a lot of energy, which means that our body will actually store the remaining carbs in our system and turn them into additional fat, which is the thing that most frequently causes weight gain. So how do we make our bodies switch to another source of energy?

Well, the most logical way to do this is to restrict the body from the source of energy that it is so used to, which are carbs. When we reduce the amount of carbs that we eat, it means that the body will burn them much faster than it was used to burning them before, which means that it will have no choice but to switch to fat as a new source of energy. Note though that this is not something that happens instantly. Depending on the kind of lifestyle that you were leading prior to you decision to switch to a Ketogenic Diet, it could take anywhere between two days and four days for the entire Ketogenic effect to take place. This is where patience really comes in as the most important source of motivation during this initial period of transition onto this style of eating. Also, some of the most frequent problems that people experience are headaches and sudden cravings. This is precisely because the body is doing everything it can to go back to the old way of eating, because it really doesn't want to deal with the complex process that is the breakdown of fatty acids as energy sources, but if you are able to push through this short period at the beginning, the body will have no other choice but to switch to a new energy source.

After a few days have passed and all of the carbohydrate sources have been used up, the body will switch t breaking down fatty acids into an energy source. The body needs the help of the liver in order to do this properly, but once this process had been completed, the source of energy that comes from fats is a powerful, and stable one. It is also the main reason why so many people report serious weight loss when they transfer to the Ketogenic Diet, and if they keep it up, the weight loss will be more and more visible and continuous for as long as the body has any extra weight to lose. But this isn't the only reason why the Ketogenic Diet is such a great thing overall for the entire body.

THE HEALTH BENEFITS OF THE KETOGENIC DIET

Weight loss is of course a great benefit of a healthy diet, and it has nothing to do with the traditional notions of beauty. The reason why weight loss is important is because all extra weight of the body has a negative effect on the spine and the joints of the body. It makes it very difficult for us to move properly and to live our lives on a daily basis. The less weight that our body has to deal with, the easier it is to live our daily lives. Also, the toxins that come with bad food choices also affect our minds and the way that our brains work. Our brains needs to be fed with healthy foods if they are to work properly and to stay healthy for a long time. Likewise, the introduction of wholefoods also means that our body will easily be able to get rid of cholesterol and also of any sign of diabetes, because there will not be any negative food sources that will cause this kind of trouble for our bodies. There are also numerous other health benefits such as eye health, hair, nail and skin health, and so much more.

The longer that the Ketogenic Diet is applied, the more time the body will have to regenerate itself into a better version of itself, and in turn it will make our lives easier and more pleasurable. Although the positive effects can certainly be noticed even in the first week of switching to a Ketogenic Diet, this does not mean that a single week is enough to change years of bad eating habits and other bad habits that may have been done to the body. As an individual, you still need to make sure that you continue to have your annual checkups with your doctor, and that you continue to have a variety of exercise sources so that your body can truly be in the best shape that it can possible be. We mention this because we don't want to provide a feeling where the change of diet alone will change everything negative that was done for years in the past. However, it is well-known that food certainly is a truly important factor when it comes to the health of the body and it needs to be taken seriously.

WHICH FOODS SHOULD AND SHOULD NOT BE EATEN ON THE KETOGENIC DIET?

In order to create the Ketogenic effect that is so important for this diet, the kind of food that will be eaten needs to be prepared and understood properly. Yes, there will be many foods that we are used to that need to be instantly eliminated from this diet, but it is truly all for the best in the long run. A few days of cravings are well worth the effort when you think of all the great benefits that will come with this new way of eating. Therefore, in order to make sure that everything is correctly understood about the Ketogenic Diet, here is an in-depth look at all the foods that should and should not be eaten and why.

Drink plenty of water

Although some people may think it almost annoying at this point how often they are told to drink water, there is a very important reason why this advice is crucial both in everyday life, but also when it comes to any change that you are making in your diet. It is also extremely important when it comes to transitioning onto the Ketogenic Diet, because your body will need a constant source of water to make sure that it can deal with all of the changes that are about to happen to it. Water is extremely important when it comes to digestion, when it comes to hydrating the human brain and making sure that it will work properly, and also when it comes to making sure that the body will be flushing out all do the toxins that really should no longer be part of it. This means that a good source of water will actually make the Ketogenic Diet more effective, it will help the body to get rid of the bad carbs faster, and it will also reduce the chance of those craving headaches from happening, which is something that so many people have to deal with. To do this properly, make sure that there is always a glass of water near you and try to sip on water continuously. Do not force yourself to drink huge amounts of water at a single time. Instead, make it a natural transition and one where your body will be continuously hydrated at all times.

No sugar, processed foods, grains, or fruit
These are the ingredients that have the highest levels of carbohydrates in them, and they are the main reason why a Ketogenic effect where the body switches to fat as a source of energy is slowed down. When these foods are eliminated, the body will be stopped from having its most favorite source of energy, and it will have to switch to fatty acids one way or another. This means that you must eliminate all processes foods, all desserts, snacks, and sugar, all grains, and all fruit for the time being. This is to make sure that the initial stages of the ketosis are enabled as soon as possible, so that the body can start to feel the benefits oft this diet quickly. Now, you might be thinking that fruit is in fact a healthy ingredient, so why would it be excluded from this diet? Fruit has a very high level of carbs as part of its ingredients, which means that even

a single fruit can really ruin all of the previous hard work that has been made to switch to ketosis. Now, because wholefood fruit does in fact have positive effects on the human body, controlled amounts of fruit can later be reintroduced into the diet. However, this is done after the body has already taken up most of the healthy benefits of this diet and at a time when it can afford to have a few fruits every now and them. However, the processed foods should continue to be avoided at all times, because they truly have no benefit for the human body and should not be consumed at any time. For those people who find themselves continue to crave some fast foods or dessert options, there are plenty of Ketogenic versions of these recipes that can be made, which will ensure that you can treat yourself every now and then without disrupting your body.

A lot of protein – from all sources

All protein sources are great for the Ketogenic Diet because they all have healthy sources of fat which will continue to be a great source of energy during this lifestyle change. Of course, this includes the fact that the source of protein need to be ones of the highest quality possible, and prepared in organic ways. Some of the best sources of protein to take inspiration from are pork, poultry, beef, fish, eggs, and seafood. Basically, any source of protein that you really enjoy eating is a great choice. When it comes to the fat content that comes from these ingredients, although you can take away any extra fat that you don't want to include in your recipe, remember that it is this far that will really help your body in the long run. One other important thing to remember is that you need to make sure that you are familiar with where your protein sources are actually coming from. If possible, choose organic options from animals that have lived an organic life on a farm, and not animals that have been force fed to grow larger at a faster rate. Poor sources of protein will have very negative effects on your body and will cause the inclusion of toxins in your diet, which remember are the things that we really want to get rid of.

Plenty of vegetables – especially leafy greens

Vegetables are extremely important for the Ketogenic Diet because they are an important source of vitamins and minerals that will help the body to run properly and to have the right energy levels that you need for your daily tasks. The best choices are spinach, kale, beans, radishes, spring onions, herbs, and beans. These are the ingredients that have the lowest number of carbs in them, or in some cases none at all. However, this does not mean that other sources of vegetables should be avoided, even if they have a higher levels of carbs. This includes vegetables such as carrots, sweet potatoes, potatoes, and red onions. They may have a higher levels of carbs in them, but it is certainly not enough to ruin the ketosis that you are aiming for, and they should be eaten in moderation. Your body still needs the energy source that it needs to run properly. As long as your energy sources are wholefoods, your body will find a way to make itself feel better.

THE BEST WAYS TO COOK FOOD ON THE KETOGENIC DIET

Now that you know the kinds of foods that are allowed and not allowed on the Ketogenic Diet, it is a good idea to go over some of the ways that these foods can be prepared. It will help you to choose the cooking styles that are most suitable for your lifestyle and your food taste, and it will also ensure that you have all the information that you need to make sure that you are preparing your food in the best way possible.

Whenever possible, do not fry your food in large amount of oil. Yes, oil may technically be classified as fat, but it is not necessarily a healthy source of fat, especially not oil that is brought to very high temperatures. Instead, consider baking your food, boiling it, or cooking it in a hot pot or an air cooker. All of these coking methods will ensure that your food will retain as many of its nutritional properties that it can possibly retain, which is of course important for keeping your body healthy. Also, avoid ordering takeaways or eating out whenever possible. Even if the food is marked as food that is suitable for a Ketogenic Diet, you can never really be sure how someone else has prepared their food or where the ingredients come from. Luckily, there are certainly great Ketogenic choices that can be made when you decide to eat out, but it is still a much better idea to make this a rare occasion rather than something that you have decided to do on a regular basis. Although the beginning may be difficult, the more you focus on making the most of the starting stages of your ketosis journey, the better the results will be in the end.

DAY-1 BREAKFAST

Delicious Mexican Frittata

Serves: 6 Preparation time: 10 minutes Cooking time: 20 minutes

8 eggs, scrambled
½ cup cheddar cheese, grated
3 scallions, chopped
13 lb tomatoes, sliced
1 small green pepper, chopped
½ cup salsa
2 tsp taco seasoning
½ lb ground beef

1 tbsp olive oil

¼ tsp salt

- Preheat the oven to 190 C 375 F.
- Heat olive oil in a medium pan over medium heat. Add ground beef and sauté until brown. Add salsa and taco seasoning and stir well to coat.
- Remove meat from the pan and place on a plate.
- Add green pepper to the pan and cook for few minutes, until crisp.
- Return meat to the pan along with scallions and tomato.
- Add scrambled eggs on top then sprinkle with grated cheese.
- Bake in preheated oven for 20-25 minutes.
- Serve warm and enjoy.

Per Serving: Net Carbs: 3.3g; Calories: 229 Total Fat: 13.8g; Saturated Fat: 5.1g Protein: 22g; Carbs: 4.4g; Fiber: 1.1g; Sugar: 2.4g; Fat 55% Protein 39% Carbs 6%

DAY-1 LUNCH

Tasty Chicken Guacamole Salad

Serves: 03 Preparation time: 15 minutes Cooking time: 10 minutes

2 chicken breasts, cooked and cubed
2 serrano chili peppers, chopped
½ cup celery, chopped
½ cup onion, chopped

1 cup cilantro, chopped
1 tbsp fresh lime juice
2 avocados, peeled and pitted
1 tsp kosher salt
Lettuce leaves for serving

- In a bowl, mash avocados with lime juice using a fork.

- Add Serrano chili peppers, onion, cilantro, and salt and stir well to combine.
- Add chicken and fold well.
- Serve salad with lettuce leaves and enjoy.

Per Serving: Net Carbs: 2.4g; Calories: 240; Total Fat: 10.6g; Saturated Fat: 2.7g Protein: 29.3g; Carbs: 5.2g; Fiber: 2.8g; Sugar: 1.1g; Fat 42% Protein 51% Carbs 7%

DAY-1 DINNER

Flavorful Chicken Piccata

Serves: 4 Preparation time: 15 minutes Cooking time: 15 minutes

8 chicken thighs, skinless and boneless
2 tbsp fresh parsley, chopped
1 tbsp butter
1 ½ tbsp fresh lemon juice
¾ cup chicken stock
1 thyme sprig
3 garlic cloves, crushed
2 tbsp capers, drained
½ cup dry white wine
3 tbsp olive oil
¼ tsp black pepper
½ tsp kosher salt

- Season chicken with pepper and salt.
- Heat 1 tablespoon of oil in a pan over medium-high heat.
- Add chicken to the pan and cook for 5 minutes.
- Turn chicken to another side. Add thyme, garlic, capers, and wine and cook for 2 minutes.
- Add stock and remaining oil to the pan. Bring to boil. Turn heat to medium and cook for 8 minutes.
- Remove pan from heat. Add butter and lemon juice. Stir well.
- Garnish with parsley and serve.

Per Serving: Net Carbs: 1.9g; Calories: 703; Total Fat: 35.3g; Saturated Fat: 9.4g Protein: 85g; Carbs: 2.2g; Fiber: 0.3g; Sugar: 0.5g; Fat 47% Protein 51% Carbs 2%

DAY-2 BREAKFAST

Healthy Egg Breakfast Muffins

Serves: 6 Preparation time: 15 minutes Cooking time: 25 minutes

12 eggs

½ cup fresh spinach, shredded

1 cup cheddar cheese, shredded

¼ cup mushrooms, chopped and sautéed

¼ cup bell pepper, diced

¼ tsp garlic powder

1 cup ham, diced and cooked

2 tbsp onion, chopped

¼ tsp black pepper

½ tsp salt

- Preheat the oven to 176 C 350 F.
- Spray 12 cup muffin pan with cooking spray and set aside.
- In a large bowl, beat eggs until well combined.
- Add remaining ingredients to the bowl and mix well together.
- Pour muffin mixture into the prepared muffin tray and bake in preheated oven for 20-25 minutes or until muffin is completely cooked from center.
- Serve and enjoy.

Per Serving: Net Carbs: 2.2g; Calories: 243 Total Fat: 17g; Saturated Fat: 7.4g Protein: 19.8g; Carbs: 2.8g; Fiber: 0.6g; Sugar: 1.3g; Fat 63% Protein 33% Carbs 4%

DAY-2 LUNCH

Creamy Cheesy Cauliflower Mash

Serves: 2 Preparation time: 10 minutes Cooking time: 15 minutes

1 cauliflower head, wash and trim
2 oz cheddar cheese, shredded
1 tbsp butter
2 tbsp heavy cream
¼ tsp black pepper
Salt

- Cut cauliflower into the medium size pieces.
- Add cauliflower, butter, and heavy cream in a microwave-safe dish and microwave on high for 6 minutes.

- Stir cauliflower until well coated with cream and butter mixture and microwave for another 6 minutes.
- Transfer cauliflower mixture into the food processor along with shredded cheddar cheese and process until smooth.
- Season with pepper and salt.
- Serve and enjoy.

Per Serving: Net Carbs: 4.5g; Calories: 250; Total Fat: 20.8g; Saturated Fat: 13.1g Protein: 10.1g; Carbs: 7.8g; Fiber: 3.3g; Sugar: 3.4g; Fat 76% Protein 17% Carbs 7%

DAY-2 DINNER

Cauliflower Cheese Casserole

Serves: 6 Preparation time: 10 minutes Cooking time: 15 minutes

1 large cauliflower head, cut into florets
1 tsp garlic powder
2 cups cheddar cheese, shredded
2 tsp Dijon mustard
2 oz cream cheese
1 cup heavy cream
½ tsp salt

- Preheat the oven to 190 C 375 F.
- Spray 9*9 baking dish with cooking spray and set aside.
- Bring large saucepan of water to boil. Add cauliflower florets and salt and cook until tender.

- Drain cauliflower florets well and place in large bowl. Set aside.
- In a small saucepan, add heavy cream and bring to simmer, stir well.
- Add Dijon mustard and cream cheese and whisk until thickens.
- Remove saucepan from heat. Add 1 cup shredded cheddar cheese and seasonings. Stir well.
- Pour saucepan mixture over cauliflower and stir gently to combine.
- Pour cauliflower mixture into the prepared baking dish and sprinkle with remaining cheese.
- Bake in preheated oven for 15 minutes.
- Serve warm and enjoy.

Per Serving: Net Carbs: 5.5g; Calories: 291; Total Fat: 23.4g; Saturated Fat: 14.7g Protein: 13.4g; Carbs: 9.1g; Fiber: 3.6g; Sugar: 3.7g; Fat 73% Protein 19% Carbs 8%

DAY-3 BREAKFAST

Jalapeno Muffins

Serves: 12 Preparation time: 10 minutes Cooking time: 20 minutes

9 eggs
1 jalapeno pepper, sliced
9 oz cheddar cheese, shredded
8 bacon slices, cooked and chopped
¾ cup heavy cream
Pepper
Salt

- Preheat the oven to 176 C 350 F.
- Spray 12 cups muffin tray with cooking spray and add cooked bacon slices to each muffin cup.
- In a large bowl, whisk together eggs, shredded cheese, cream, pepper, and salt.
- Pour egg mixture into the prepared muffin cups evenly.
- Now add sliced jalapeno into each muffin cup.
- Bake in preheated oven for 15-20 minutes.
- Serve and enjoy.

Per Serving: Net Carbs: 1g; Calories: 236 Total Fat: 19.1g; Saturated Fat: 9.2g Protein: 14.9g; Carbs: 1g; Fiber: 0g; Sugar: 0.4g; Fat 73% Protein 25% Carbs 2%

DAY-3 LUNCH

Bacon Avocado Chicken Salad

Serves: 4 Preparation time: 10 minutes Cooking time: 10 minutes

2 chicken breasts, cooked and chopped
3 tbsp olive oil
3 tbsp fresh lemon juice
1 tsp dried dill
1 tbsp dried chives
4 bacon slices, cooked and chopped
1 cup celery, diced
2 avocado, chopped
½ tsp black pepper
1 tsp salt

- Add all ingredients large mixing bowl and toss well to combine.

- Serve and enjoy.

Per Serving: Net Carbs: 2.9g; Calories: 545; Total Fat: 43.6g; Saturated Fat: 9.8g Protein: 30.4g; Carbs: 10.2g; Fiber: 7.3g; Sugar: 1.1g; Fat 73% Protein 23% Carbs 4%

DAY-3 DINNER

Perfect Bacon Chicken

Serves: 6 Preparation time: 10 minutes Cooking time: 40 minutes

6 chicken breasts, cut in half
4 oz cheddar cheese, shredded
½ lb bacon, cut into strips
2 tbsp smoked paprika rub

- Preheat the oven to 204 C 400 F.
- Spray large baking tray with cooking spray and set aside.
- Rub chicken breasts from both the sides with smoked paprika rub and place in prepared baking tray.
- Top each chicken breast with bacon slice and bake in preheated oven for 30 minutes.

- After 30 minutes remove baking tray from oven and sprinkle shredded cheese on top of chicken and bacon.
- Return chicken in oven and bake for 10 minutes more or until cheese is bubbly.
- Serve and enjoy.

Per Serving: Net Carbs: 1.2g; Calories: 565; Total Fat: 33.2g; Saturated Fat: 12.2g Protein: 61.3g; Carbs: 2.1g; Fiber: 0.9g; Sugar: 0.3g; Fat 53% Protein 45% Carbs 2%

DAY-4 BREAKFAST

Easy Breakfast Bowl

Serves: 1 Preparation time: 5 minutes Cooking time: 15 minutes

2 eggs
½ cup cheddar cheese, shredded
3 bacon strips, cooked and crumbled
½ avocado, sliced

2 tbsp butter

Pepper

Salt

- Melt butter in a pan over medium heat.
- Add eggs into the pan and cook until scrambled. Season with pepper and salt.
- Transfer scrambled egg into the soup bowl.
- Add shredded cheese on top of scramble eggs.
- Top with bacon and avocado slices.
- Serve and enjoy.

Per Serving: Net Carbs: 1.6g; Calories: 603 Total Fat: 54.5g; Saturated Fat: 30g Protein: 26.4g; Carbs: 3.2g; Fiber: 1.6g; Sugar: 1g; Fat 81% Protein 18% Carbs 1%

DAY-4 LUNCH

Creamy Egg Salad

Serves: 4 Preparation time: 15 minutes Cooking time: 10 minutes

8 eggs, boiled
23 cup mayonnaise
1 tsp yellow mustard
1 green pepper, chopped
2 green onion, chopped
2 celery stalks, chopped
Pepper
Salt

- Peeled and chopped boiled eggs.
- In a mixing bowl, mix together mustard and mayonnaise.
- Add remaining ingredients and stir well to combine.

- Season salad with pepper and salt.
- Serve and enjoy.

Per Serving: Net Carbs: 5.3g; Calories: 266; Total Fat: 22.1g; Saturated Fat: 4.8g Protein: 11.9g; Carbs: 6.2g; Fiber: 0.9g; Sugar: 3.4g; Fat 75% Protein 18% Carbs 7%

DAY-4 DINNER

Quick Cherry Tomato Frittata

Serves: 2 Preparation time: 10 minutes Cooking time: ## minutes

6 eggs
1 tbsp chives, chopped
1 tbsp basil, chopped
1 tbsp butter
23 cup cherry tomatoes, halved
23 cup feta cheese, crumbled
½ onion, sliced
Pepper
Salt

- Preheat the oven to 204 C 400 F.
- Melt butter in a pan over medium heat.

- Add sliced onion to the pan and sauté until lightly browned.
- In a bowl, whisk eggs with chives, basil, pepper, and salt.
- Once onion is lightly browned then add egg mixture and cook for 2-3 minutes.
- Top with crumbled feta cheese and cherry tomatoes. Place in preheated oven and cook for 5-7 minutes.
- Serve and enjoy.

Per Serving: Net Carbs: 6.7g; Calories: 394; Total Fat: 29.7g; Saturated Fat: 15.2g Protein: 24.7g; Carbs: 8.1g; Fiber: 1.4g; Sugar: 5.9g; Fat 68% Protein 25% Carbs 7%

DAY-5 BREAKFAST

Egg Breakfast Casserole

Serves: 8 Preparation time: 10 minutes Cooking time: 35 minutes

10 eggs

¼ cup goat cheese, crumbled
4 cherry tomatoes, halved
13 cup cheddar cheese, grated
13 cup ham
1 small zucchini, sliced
½ cup spinach
23 cup heavy cream
Pepper
Salt

- Preheat the oven to 176 C 350 F.
- Spray 9*13 baking pan with cooking spray and set aside.
- Whisk eggs in a bowl with cream, pepper, and salt.
- Add cheddar cheese, ham, zucchini, and spinach and stir well.
- Pour egg mixture into the prepared pan and top with cherry tomatoes and goat cheese.
- Bake in preheated oven for 30-35 minutes.
- Remove from oven and set aside to cool completely.
- Serve and enjoy.

Per Serving: Net Carbs: 3.7g; Calories: 169 Total Fat: 12.3g; Saturated Fat: 5.6g Protein: 10.5g; Carbs: 4.6g; Fiber: 0.9g; Sugar: 1.9g; Fat 66% Protein 25% Carbs 9%

DAY-5 LUNCH

Chicken Basil Salad

Serves: 1 Preparation time: 10 minutes Cooking time: 5 minutes

1 cup chicken breast, cooked and shredded

1 tsp vinegar

1 tbsp sour cream

2 tsp fresh basil, chopped

¼ cup cucumber, diced

Pepper

Salt

- Add all ingredients into the mixing bowl and toss well to combine.
- Season salad with pepper and salt.
- Place in refrigerator for 10 minutes.
- Serve chilled and enjoy.

Per Serving: Net Carbs: 1.4g; Calories: 243; Total Fat: 6.8g; Saturated Fat: 2.8g

Protein: 41.2g; Carbs: 1.6g; Fiber: 0.2g; Sugar: 0.5g; Fat 27% Protein 69% Carbs 4%

DAY-5 DINNER

Smoked Paprika Chicken

Serves: 4 Preparation time: 10 minutes Cooking time: ## minutes

4 chicken breasts, skinless and boneless, cut into chunks
2 tsp garlic, minced
2 tbsp lemon juice
2 tbsp smoked paprika
3 tbsp olive oil
Pepper
Salt

- Preheat the oven to 176 C 350 F.
- In a small bowl, mix together garlic, lemon juice, paprika, and olive oil.
- Season chicken with pepper and salt.

- Spread 13 bowl mixture on the bottom of casserole dish.
- Add seasoned chicken into the casserole dish and rub with dish sauce.
- Pour remaining sauce on top of chicken and rub well.
- Bake in preheated oven for 30-35 minutes.
- Serve and enjoy.

Per Serving: Net Carbs: 1.2g; Calories: 381; Total Fat: 21.8g; Saturated Fat: 4.6g Protein: 42.9g; Carbs: 2.6g; Fiber: 1.4g; Sugar: 0.5g; Fat 53% Protein 45% Carbs 2%

DAY-6 BREAKFAST

Almond Blueberry Muffins

Serves: 12 Preparation time: 10 minutes Cooking time: 20 minutes

3 eggs
¾ cup blueberries

½ tsp vanilla

13 cup unsweetened almond milk

13 cup coconut oil, melted

1 ½ tsp baking powder, gluten free

½ cup erythritol

2 ½ cups almond flour

¼ tsp sea salt

- Preheat the oven to 176 C 350 F.
- Line muffin tray with muffin liners and set aside.
- In a large mixing bowl, mix together almond flour, baking powder, erythritol, and sea salt.
- Add eggs, vanilla, almond milk, and coconut oil and mix well.
- Add blueberries and fold well.
- Pour batter into the prepared muffin tray and bake in preheated oven for 20 minutes.
- Serve and enjoy.

Per Serving: Net Carbs: 2.1g; Calories: 109 Total Fat: 10.2g; Saturated Fat: 5.8g Protein: 2.7g; Carbs: 3g; Fiber: 0.9g; Sugar: 1.2g; Fat 84% Protein 9% Carbs 7%

DAY-6 LUNCH

Mayo Shrimp Cilantro Salad

Serves: 4 Preparation time: 15 minutes Cooking time: 10 minutes

1 lb medium shrimp, peeled, deveined, and cooked
2 tbsp fresh lime juice
1 jalapeno pepper, chopped
4 tbsp mayonnaise
2 hard-boiled eggs, chopped
½ green bell pepper, chopped
2 celery stalks, diced
2 radishes, diced
½ onion, diced
Salt

- Add all ingredients into the large mixing bowl and toss well to combine.
- Serve immediately and enjoy.

Per Serving: Net Carbs: 5.9g; Calories: 192; Total Fat: 8.2g; Saturated Fat: 1.4g Protein: 19.3g; Carbs: 6.2g; Fiber: 0.8g; Sugar: 2.7g; Fat 41% Protein 43% Carbs 16%

DAY-6 DINNER

Simple Coconut Shrimp

Serves: 4 Preparation time: 10 minutes Cooking time: 10 minutes

1 lb shrimp, deveined

½ cup unsweetened coconut milk

1 tsp garam masala

½ tsp cayenne pepper

½ tsp turmeric

1 tbsp garlic, minced

1 tbsp ginger, minced

1 tsp salt

- Add all ingredients into the saucepan and stir well.
- Heat saucepan over medium heat until shrimp is cooked.
- Stir well and serve with cauliflower rice.

Per Serving: Net Carbs: 4.3g; Calories: 213; Total Fat: 9.2g; Saturated Fat: 7g

Protein: 26.8g; Carbs: 5.3g; Fiber:1 g; Sugar: 1.1g; Fat 40% Protein 51% Carbs 9%

DAY-7 BREAKFAST

Cheddar Broccoli Bread

Serves: 10 Preparation time: 10 minutes Cooking time: 30 minutes

5 eggs, lightly beaten

2 tsp baking powder, gluten free

3 12 tbsp coconut flour

¾ cup broccoli, chopped

1 cup cheddar cheese, shredded

1 tsp salt

- Preheat the oven to 176 C 350 F.
- Spray loaf pan with cooking spray and set aside.
- In a mixing bowl, add all ingredients and whisk until well combined.
- Pour egg mixture into the prepared loaf pan.
- Bake in preheated oven for 30-35 minutes.
- Cut into the slices and serve.

Per Serving: Net Carbs: 2g; Calories: 101 Total Fat: 6.7g; Saturated Fat: 3.8g

Protein: 6.5g; Carbs: 4g; Fiber: 2g; Sugar: 0.7g; Fat 62% Protein 28% Carbs 10%

DAY-7 LUNCH

Flavorful Tuna Salad

Serves: 8 Preparation time: 10 minutes Cooking time: 10 minutes

3 cans tuna, drained and flaked
2 tbsp olive oil
½ lemon juice
¼ cup cilantro, chopped
½ onion, sliced
3 medium avocados, peeled, pitted, and chopped
2 large celery stalks, diced
18 tsp pepper
1 tsp sea salt

- Add all ingredients into the large mixing bowl and toss well to combine.
- Serve and enjoy.

Per Serving: Net Carbs: 0.8g; Calories: 183; Total Fat: 10.8g;   Saturated   Fat: 2g

Protein: 18.3g; Carbs: 2.4g; Fiber: 1.6g; Sugar: 0.6g; Fat 55% Protein 42% Carbs 3%

DAY-7 DINNER

Tuna Egg Bake

Serves: 8   Preparation time: 15 minutes   Cooking time: 45 minutes

6 eggs
½ tsp dried chilies
½ tsp garlic powder
½ tsp cayenne
½ cup coconut milk
¼ tsp sea salt
For filling:
1 can tuna, drained
2 cups spring greens, chopped
1 bell pepper, diced
2 mushrooms, sliced
1 medium onion, diced
½ tsp pepper
¼ tsp sea salt

- Preheat the oven to 176 C 350 F.

- In a large bowl, whisk together eggs, coconut milk, dried chilies, sea salt, garlic powder, and cayenne.
- Spray oven safe pan with cooking spray and heat over medium heat.
- Add mushroom and onion to the pan and sauté until soften.
- Add bell peppers and cook for 4 minutes more.
- Add spring green and cook until wilted.
- Add tuna and stir until well combined.
- Now add egg mixture. Place in preheated oven and cook for 40-45 minutes.
- Serve and enjoy.

Per Serving: Net Carbs: 3.1g; Calories: 138; Total Fat: 8.8g; Saturated Fat: 4.6g Protein: 11.1g; Carbs: 4.4g; Fiber: 1.3g; Sugar: 2.3g; Fat 58% Protein 33% Carbs 9%

DAY-8 BREAKFAST

Delicious Ricotta Omelet

Serves: 1 Preparation time: 10 minutes Cooking time: 10 minutes

3 eggs

2 tbsp sun-dried tomatoes, chopped

2 tbsp mozzarella cheese, shredded

1 tbsp fresh basil, chopped

2 tbsp ricotta whole milk

1 tsp butter

- Melt butter in a pan over medium heat.
- Meanwhile, in a bowl, whisk together eggs, sun-dried tomatoes, and basil.
- Pour egg mixture into the pan. Cover pan with lid and cook over medium-low heat.
- Mix together mozzarella cheese and ricotta.
- Remove pan lid and add mozzarella mixture on top of omelet.
- Cover pan again and cook for 1-2 minutes or until omelet cooked through.
- Transfer omelet onto a serving plate and fold it and serve.

Per Serving: Net Carbs: 4.6g; Calories: 441 Total Fat: 31g; Saturated Fat: 15.1g

Protein: 36.4g; Carbs: 4.9g; Fiber: 0.3g; Sugar: 1.7g; Fat 63% Protein 33% Carbs 4%

DAY-8 LUNCH

Flavorful Citrusy Shrimp

Serves: 3 Preparation time: 10 minutes Cooking time: 10 minutes

1 lb shrimp
1 tbsp fresh parsley, chopped
1 tsp lemon zest
1 tbsp fresh lemon juice
3 garlic cloves, minced
2 tbsp olive oil
½ tsp black pepper
½ tsp sea salt

- Season shrimp with pepper and salt.
- Heat olive oil in a pan over medium heat.
- Add garlic to the pan and sauté until brown.
- Add shrimp and sauté for 1 minute.
- Add lemon zest and lemon juice and stir well. Cook shrimp over medium heat until cooked through.
- Garnish with parsley and serve.

Per Serving: Net Carbs: 3.6g; Calories: 267; Total Fat: 12g; Saturated Fat: 2.2g Protein: 34.8g; Carbs: 3.9g; Fiber: 0.3g; Sugar: 0.2g; Fat 41% Protein 53% Carbs 6%

DAY-8 DINNER

Simple Old Bay Seasoned Shrimp

Serves: 1   Preparation time: 5 minutes   Cooking time: 10 minutes

32 oz shrimp, peeled and deveined
½ lemon juice
2 tbsp old bay seasoning
1 tbsp olive oil

- Add all ingredients into the large bowl and toss until well coated.
- Heat large pan over medium-high heat.
- Add shrimp into the pan and cook for 2 minutes on each side.
- Serve with zoodles and enjoy.

Per Serving: Net Carbs: 3.6g; Calories: 301; Total Fat: 7.4g; Saturated Fat: 1.7g Protein: 51.7g; Carbs: 3.6g; Fiber: 0g; Sugar: 0.1g; Fat 24% Protein 70% Carbs 6%

DAY-9 BREAKFAST

Olive Bacon Quiche

Serves: 8 Preparation time: 10 minutes Cooking time: 30 minutes

12 eggs, whisked
¾ cup coconut cream
3 garlic cloves, minced
¼ cup fresh basil leaves
15 olives, diced
2 small tomatoes, diced
4 cups spinach, chopped
1 onion, diced
2 bell peppers, diced
6 bacon slices, diced
3 tbsp coconut oil
Pepper
Salt

- Preheat the oven 176 C 350 F.
- Melt coconut oil in a large pan over medium-high heat.
- Add bacon and cook for 3-4 minutes or until crispy. Remove from pan and set aside.

- Add onion and bell pepper in same pan and sauté for 5 minutes.
- Add spinach and sauté for 1-2 minutes.
- Remove pan from heat and set aside.
- In a large mixing bowl, mix together eggs, bacon, coconut cream, garlic, basil, olives, tomato, and spinach mixture. Season with pepper and salt.
- Pour egg mixture into the 9" baking dish and bake in preheated oven for 30 minutes.
- Serve and enjoy.

Per Serving: Net Carbs: 5.7g; Calories: 301 Total Fat: 24.1g; Saturated Fat: 13.3g Protein: 15.3g; Carbs: 7.8g; Fiber: 2.1g; Sugar: 4g; Fat 72% Protein 20% Carbs 8%

DAY-9 LUNCH

Easy Cabbage Noodles

Serves: 4 Preparation time: 10 minutes Cooking time: 10 minutes

1 lb cabbage, cored and cut into strips

2 tbsp butter

2 garlic cloves, sliced

¼ cup onion, sliced

Pepper

Salt

- Melt butter in a pan over medium heat.
- Add garlic, onion, and cabbage and sauté for 10 minutes or until cabbage is tender.
- Season with pepper and salt.
- Serve and enjoy.

Per Serving: Net Carbs: 4.8g; Calories: 84; Total Fat: 5.9g; Saturated Fat: 3.7g Protein: 1.7g; Carbs: 7.8g; Fiber: 3g; Sugar: 4g; Fat 65% Protein 10% Carbs 25%

DAY-9 DINNER

Cauliflower Cheese Casserole

Serves: 8 Preparation time: 15 minutes Cooking time: 30 minutes

6 tbsp fresh chives, chopped

1 cup cheddar cheese, shredded

1 cup Monterey jack cheese, shredded

1 tbsp ranch seasoning

½ cup mayonnaise

½ cup sour cream

1 large head cauliflower, cut into florets

8 bacon slices, cooked and crumbled

¼ tsp pepper

- Preheat the oven to 187 C 370 F.
- Spray 13*9 baking dish with cooking spray and set aside.
- Steam cauliflower florets for 15-20 minutes or until tender.
- In a large bowl, combine together sour cream, ranch seasoning, mayonnaise, and black pepper.

- Add steam cauliflower, 3 tbsp chives, 1 cup cheddar cheese, and half of bacon into the bowl and mix well.
- Pour mixture into the prepared baking dish and top with Monterey jack cheese and remaining bacon.
- Cover dish with foil and bake in preheated oven for 20 minutes.
- Remove foil and bake for 10 minutes more.
- Garnish with remaining chives and serve.

Per Serving: Net Carbs: 4.2g; Calories: 364; Total Fat: 30g; Saturated Fat: 11.7g Protein: 16.6g; Carbs: 6.9g; Fiber: 2.7g; Sugar: 2.7g; Fat 75% Protein 19% Carbs 6%

DAY-10 BREAKFAST

Coconut Waffles

Serves: 4 Preparation time: 10 minutes Cooking time: 10 minutes

4 eggs
1 ½ tsp baking powder
4 tbsp coconut flour
1 tbsp powdered stevia
1 tsp vanilla
1 tbsp butter, melted
4 oz cream cheese

- Preheat the waffle iron.
- Add all ingredients into the blender and blend until smooth.
- Spray waffle iron with cooking spray.
- Pour ¼ cup batter for each waffle in hot waffle maker and cook according to the waffle iron instructions.
- Serve and enjoy.

Per Serving: Net Carbs: 3.6g; Calories: 227 Total Fat: 18.4g; Saturated Fat: 10.4g Protein: 9.2g; Carbs: 6.6g; Fiber: 3g; Sugar: 1g; Fat 74% Protein 18% Carbs 8%

DAY-10 LUNCH

Curried Chicken Salad

Serves: 4 Preparation time: 10 minutes Cooking time: 10 minutes

2 oz walnuts, chopped

2 tbsp green onion, chopped

8 oz chicken, cooked and diced

For dressing:

2 tbsp fresh cilantro, chopped

18 tsp cayenne

1 tsp curry powder

1 tbsp lemon juice

½ cup mayonnaise

¼ tsp pepper

¼ tsp salt

- In a small bowl, mix together all dressing ingredients and set aside.
- Add walnuts, green onion, and chicken into the large mixing bowl and mix well.
- Pour dressing over salad and toss well to coat.
- Serve and enjoy.

Per Serving: Net Carbs: 0.9g; Calories: 372; Total Fat: 31.5g; Saturated Fat: 4.7g Protein: 18.6g; Carbs: 2.4g; Fiber: 1.5g; Sugar: 0.5g; Fat 78% Protein 20% Carbs 2%

DAY-10 DINNER

Cheese Broccoli Soup

Serves: 8 Preparation time: 10 minutes Cooking time: 15 minutes

4 cups broccoli, cut into florets

3 1⁄2 cups vegetable broth

2 garlic cloves, minced

1 tbsp olive oil

3 cups cheddar cheese, shredded

1 cup heavy cream

Pepper

Salt

- Heat olive oil in a large pot over medium heat.
- Add garlic and sauté for a minute.
- Add broth, broccoli, and heavy cream and bring to boil, reduce heat and simmer for 15 minutes.
- Add shredded cheese and stir continuously until cheese is melted.
- Season with pepper and salt.
- Remove from heat and serve.

Per Serving: Net Carbs: 3.4g; Calories: 271; Total Fat: 22.1g; Saturated Fat: 12.8g Protein: 14.3g; Carbs: 4.6g; Fiber: 1.2g; Sugar: 1.3g; Fat 73% Protein 22% Carbs 5%

DAY-11 BREAKFAST

Easy Egg Loaf

Serves: 4   Preparation time: 5 minutes   Cooking time: 30 minutes

4 eggs

1 tsp swerve

1 tsp vanilla

4 oz cream cheese

4 tbsp butter

- Add all ingredients into the small bowl and mix with electric mixer until well combined and smooth.
- Spray 9*13 baking pan with cooking spray.
- Pour batter into the prepared pan and bake at 176 C 350 F for 30 minutes.
- Serve and enjoy.

Per Serving: Net Carbs: 1.7g; Calories: 268 Total Fat: 25.8g; Saturated Fat: 14.9g Protein: 7.8g; Carbs: 1.7g; Fiber: 0g; Sugar: 0.5g; Fat 86% Protein 12% Carbs 2%

DAY-11 LUNCH

Almond Chicken Salad

Serves: 2 Preparation time: 15 minutes Cooking time: 5 minutes

2 cups chicken breasts, cooked and diced

1 tsp curry powder

2 medium celery stalks, chopped

2 tbsp almonds, chopped

¼ cup mayonnaise

Salt

- Add all ingredients into the large bowl and toss well to combine.
- Serve and enjoy.

Per Serving: Net Carbs: 1.3g; Calories: 490; Total Fat: 33.6g; Saturated Fat: 6.1g Protein: 42.2g; Carbs: 3g; Fiber: 1.7g; Sugar: 0.8g; Fat 63% Protein 35% Carbs 2%

DAY-11 DINNER

Shrimp Mushroom Soup

Serves: 8 Preparation time: 10 minutes Cooking time: 15 minutes

24 oz shrimp, cooked
32 oz chicken broth
2 cups mushrooms, sliced
8 oz cheddar cheese, shredded
½ cup butter
1 cup heavy whipping cream
Pepper
Salt

- Add broth and mushrooms to a large pot. Bring to boil over high heat.
- Turn heat to medium and add cheese, whipping cream, and butter and stir until cheese is melted.
- Reduce heat and add shrimp. Stir well and cook for 2 minutes more.
- Serve and enjoy.

Per Serving: Net Carbs: 2.9g; Calories: 391; Total Fat: 28.6g; Saturated Fat: 17.3g Protein: 29.7g; Carbs: 3.1g; Fiber: 0.2g; Sugar: 0.8g; Fat 66% Protein 31% Carbs 3%

DAY-12 BREAKFAST

Delicious Breakfast Cookies

Serves: 8 Preparation time: 10 minutes Cooking time: 25 minutes

3 eggs

1 cup cheddar cheese, shredded

6 bacon slices, cooked and crumbled

¼ lb sausage, cooked and crumbled

½ tsp garlic powder

2 tsp baking powder

6 tbsp coconut flour

8 oz cream cheese, softened

½ tsp black pepper

¾ tsp salt

- Preheat the oven to 176 C 350 F.
- Spray baking tray with cooking spray and line with parchment paper. Set aside.
- In a large bowl, beat together eggs and cream cheese until smooth.
- Add coconut flour, garlic powder, baking powder, pepper and salt and beat until well combined.
- Add cheese, bacon, and sausage and stir well.
- Spoon cookie mixture into eight mounds onto a prepared baking tray and using hands press down to 1 inch thickness.
- Bake in preheated oven for 20-25 minutes or until lightly golden brown.
- Remove from oven and set aside to cool completely.
- Serve and enjoy.

Per Serving: Net Carbs: 3.1g; Calories: 329 Total Fat: 26.9g; Saturated Fat: 13.7g Protein: 16.6g; Carbs: 5.1g; Fiber: 2g; Sugar: 0.7g; Fat 72% Protein 25% Carbs 3%

DAY-12 LUNCH

Cucumber Tuna Salad

Serves: 2 Preparation time: 10 minutes Cooking time: 5 minutes

2 cans tuna water packed

½ lime juice

13 cup mayonnaise

½ cucumber, peeled and chopped

¼ small onion, chopped

1 celery stalk, chopped

Pepper

Salt

- Add all ingredients into the mixing bowl and mix until well combined.
- Serve and enjoy.

Per Serving: Net Carbs: 4.4g; Calories: 592; Total Fat: 41.2g; Saturated Fat: 7g Protein: 48g; Carbs: 5.6g; Fiber: 1.2g; Sugar: 2g; Fat 63% Protein 34% Carbs 3%

DAY-12 DINNER

Delicious Ranch Chicken

Serves: 6 Preparation time: 10 minutes Cooking time: 6 hours

2 lbs chicken, skinless and boneless
3 tbsp butter
4 oz cream cheese
3 tbsp dry ranch dressing
Pepper
Salt

- Season chicken with pepper and salt and place into the slow cooker.
- Add butter and cheese over the chicken.
- Sprinkle dry ranch dressing over the chicken.
- Cover slow cooker with lid and cook on low for 6 hours.
- Shred the chicken using fork and serve.

Per Serving: Net Carbs: 0.9g; Calories: 347; Total Fat: 17g; Saturated Fat: 9.1g

Protein: 45.4g; Carbs: 0.9g; Fiber: 0g; Sugar: 0.2g; Fat 46% Protein 52% Carbs 2%

DAY-13 BREAKFAST

Bacon Cheese Bread

Serves: 10 Preparation time: 10 minutes Cooking time: 50 minutes

½ lb bacon, diced
1 cup cheddar cheese, grated
2 eggs
13 cup sour cream
4 tbsp butter, melted
1 tbsp baking powder
1 12 cups almond flour

- Preheat the oven to 150 C 300 F.
- Spray loaf pan with cooking spray and set aside.
- Cook bacon in a pan over medium heat until crispy.
- Meanwhile, in a large bowl, mix together almond flour and baking powder.
- In another bowl, whisk together eggs and sour cream until smooth.

- Pour egg mixture into the almond flour and mix until combined.
- Add cheese, bacon, and butter and fold well.
- Pour bread mixture into the prepared loaf pan and bake in preheated oven for 45-50 minutes.
- Slices and serve.

Per Serving: Net Carbs: 2g; Calories: 263 Total Fat: 22.4g; Saturated Fat: 9.8g Protein: 13.5g; Carbs: 2.5g; Fiber: 0.5g; Sugar: 0.3g; Fat 76% Protein 20% Carbs 4%

DAY-13 LUNCH

Chili Garlic Shrimp

Serves: 2 Preparation time: 10 minutes Cooking time: 10 minutes

1 lb shrimp, cooked
1 tsp cumin powder
1 tsp chili powder
2 garlic cloves, minced
½ bell pepper, chopped
3 tbsp olive oil

- Heat a large pan over medium heat.
- Add all ingredients into the pan and sauté until bell pepper are cooked.
- Serve and enjoy.

Per Serving: Net Carbs: 5.9g; Calories: 468 Total Fat: 25.4g; Saturated Fat: 4.2g Protein: 52.5g; Carbs: 7g; Fiber: 1.1g; Sugar: 0.8g; Fat 50% Protein 45% Carbs 5%

DAY-13 DINNER

Pesto Cheese Salmon

Serves: 2 Preparation time: 10 minutes Cooking time: 20 minutes

2 salmon fillets
¼ cup parmesan cheese, grated
For pesto:
2 garlic cloves, peeled and chopped
¼ cup olive oil
1 ½ cups fresh basil leaves
¼ cup parmesan cheese, grated
¼ cup pine nuts
½ tsp black pepper
½ tsp salt

- Add all pesto ingredients to the blender and blend until smooth.
- Preheat the oven to 204 C 400 F.
- Place salmon fillet on a baking tray and spread 2 tablespoons of the pesto on each salmon fillet.
- Sprinkle grated cheese on top of pesto.

- Bake in preheated oven for 20 minutes.
- Serve and enjoy.

Per Serving: Net Carbs: 2.9g; Calories: 726; Total Fat: 57g; Saturated Fat: 12g Protein: 49.7g; Carbs: 4g; Fiber: 1.1g; Sugar: 0.7g; Fat 71% Protein 28% Carbs 1%

DAY-14 BREAKFAST

Coconut Chia Pudding

Serves: 1 Preparation time: 5 minutes Cooking time: 5 minutes

2 tbsp chia seeds

¾ cup coconut milk

½ tsp vanilla

1 fresh strawberry, sliced

- Add all ingredients except strawberry into the glass jar and mix well.
- Cover jar with lid and place in refrigerator for overnight.
- Top with sliced strawberry and serve.

Per Serving: Net Carbs: 6.1g; Calories: 173 Total Fat: 13.6g; Saturated Fat: 8g Protein: 4.3g; Carbs: 6.3g; Fiber: 0.2g; Sugar: 0.9g; Fat 73% Protein 12% Carbs 15%

DAY-14 LUNCH

Avocado Bacon Soup

Serves: 4 Preparation time: 10 minutes Cooking time: 10 minutes

½ lb bacon, cooked and chopped
½ lime juice
2 avocados, pitted
1 tsp garlic powder
13 cup fresh cilantro, chopped
4 cups chicken stock
Pepper
Salt

- Add chicken stock into the saucepan and bring to boil over low heat.
- Add avocados, lime juice, garlic powder, and cilantro into the blender.
- Add 1 cup warm chicken stock into the blender and blend until smooth.
- Remove saucepan from heat.

- Add blended avocado mixture and bacon into the saucepan and stir well.
- Season soup with pepper and salt.
- Serve warm and enjoy.

Per Serving: Net Carbs: 2.4g; Calories: 351; Total Fat: 26.8g; Saturated Fat: 8.4g Protein: 22.4g; Carbs: 4.1g; Fiber: 1.7g; Sugar: 1g; Fat 70% Protein 27% Carbs 3%

DAY-14 DINNER

Lemon Parmesan Salmon

Serves: 4 Preparation time: 10 minutes Cooking time: 15 minutes

4 salmon fillets
¼ cup parmesan cheese, grated
½ cup walnuts
1 tsp olive oil
1 tbsp lemon rind

- Preheat the oven to 204 C 400 F.
- Spray a baking tray with cooking spray.
- Place salmon on a baking tray.
- Add walnuts into the food processor and process until finely ground.
- Mix ground walnuts with parmesan cheese, oil, and lemon rind. Stir well.
- Spread walnut mixture over the salmon fillets and press gently.
- Bake in preheated oven for 15 minutes.
- Serve and enjoy.

Per Serving: Net Carbs: 0.7g; Calories: 493; Total Fat: 30.4g; Saturated Fat: 8.3g Protein: 50.4g; Carbs: 1.9g; Fiber: 1.2g; Sugar: 0.3g; Fat 57% Protein 42% Carbs 1%

DAY-15 BREAKFAST

Spinach Bacon Frittata

Serves: 4 Preparation time: 10 minutes Cooking time: 30 minutes

8 eggs

5 oz cheddar cheese, shredded

1 cup heavy whipping cream

8 oz fresh spinach

2 tbsp butter

5 oz bacon, diced

Pepper

Salt

- Preheat the oven to 176 C 350 F.
- Spray 9*9 baking dish with cooking spray and set aside.
- Melt butter in a pan over medium heat.
- Add bacon in a pan and cook until crispy.
- Add spinach and cook until wilted. Remove pan from heat and set aside.
- In a bowl, whisk together heavy whipping cream and eggs.
- Pour cream and egg mixture into the prepared dish.
- Add bacon and spinach into the egg mixture and top with shredded cheddar cheese.
- Bake in preheated oven for 25-30 minutes.
- Serve and enjoy.

Per Serving: Net Carbs: 3.3g; Calories: 628 Total Fat: 52.4g; Saturated Fat: 25.7g Protein: 35.3g; Carbs: 4.6g; Fiber: 1.3g; Sugar: 1.1g; Fat 75% Protein 23% Carbs 2%

DAY-15 LUNCH

Italian Pepperoni Avocado Salad

Serves: 1 Preparation time: 5 minutes Cooking time: 5 minutes

1 oz mozzarella pearls
15 pepperoni slices
½ avocado, cubed
½ tbsp fresh lime juice
1 tsp Italian seasoning
Pepper
Salt

- Add all ingredients into the small bowl and toss well to combine.
- Serve and enjoy.

Per Serving: Net Carbs: 0.7g; Calories: 524; Total Fat: 45.2g; Saturated Fat: 16.5g Protein: 24.3g; Carbs: 2.2g; Fiber: 1.5g; Sugar: 0.4g; Fat 79% Protein 20% Carbs 1%

DAY-15 DINNER

Garlic Onion Pork Tenderloin

Serves: 6 Preparation time: 10 minutes Cooking time: 30 minutes

2 lbs pork tenderloin
For rub:
1 tbsp onion powder
1 tbsp smoked paprika
1 tbsp garlic powder
½ tbsp salt

- Preheat the oven to 218 C 425 F.
- In a small bowl, combine together all rub ingredients and rub over pork tenderloin.
- Heat oven-safe pan over medium-high heat.
- Spray pan with cooking spray. Sear pork on all sides until lightly golden brown.
- Place pan into the preheated oven and roast for about 25-30 minutes.
- Cut into slices and serve.

Per Serving: Net Carbs: 2g; Calories: 228; Total Fat: 5.5g; Saturated Fat: 1.8g Protein: 40.1g; Carbs: 2.6g; Fiber: 0.6g; Sugar: 0.9g; Fat 24% Protein 71% Carbs 5%

DAY-16 BREAKFAST

Healthy Coconut Porridge

Serves: 1   Preparation time: 5 minutes   Cooking time: 10 minutes

1 egg
4 tbsp coconut cream
1 tbsp coconut flour
1 oz coconut oil
Pinch of salt

- Add all ingredients into the small saucepan and stir well.
- Cook over low heat until get desired consistency.
- Top with fresh berries or coconut flakes.
- Serve and enjoy.

Per Serving: Net Carbs: 4.4g; Calories: 475 Total Fat: 47.8g; Saturated Fat: 39.1g Protein: 7.9g; Carbs: 8.7g; Fiber: 4.3g; Sugar: 2.3g; Fat 90% Protein 7% Carbs 3%

DAY-16 LUNCH

Cilantro Shrimp Avocado Salad

Serves: 6 Preparation time: 10 minutes Cooking time: 10 minutes

1 lb shrimp, cooked
2 cups lettuce, chopped
2 avocados, chopped
2 cups spinach
For dressing:
3 tbsp fresh lime juice
½ cup fresh cilantro, chopped
2 tbsp olive oil
18 tsp black pepper
Pinch of salt

- In a small bowl, combine together all dressing ingredients and set aside.
- Add shrimp into the large mixing bowl. Pour dressing over shrimp and toss well.
- Place shrimp in refrigerator for 1 hour.

- Add lettuce, avocados, and spinach into the shrimp and toss well.
- Serve and enjoy.

Per Serving: Net Carbs: 3.1g; Calories: 272; Total Fat: 19.1g; Saturated Fat: 3.8g Protein: 18.9g; Carbs: 8g; Fiber: 4.9g; Sugar: 0.6g; Fat 65% Protein 29% Carbs 6%

DAY-16 DINNER

Lemon Garlic Chicken

Serves: 4 Preparation time: 10 minutes Cooking time: 40 minutes

2 lbs chicken drumsticks

1 fresh lemon juice

10 garlic cloves, sliced

2 tbsp olive oil

4 tbsp butter

2 tbsp parsley, chopped

Pepper

Salt

- Preheat the oven to 225 C 450 F.
- Grease baking tray with butter then place chicken pieces in butter greased pan.
- Season chicken with pepper and salt.
- Sprinkle the parsley and garlic over the chicken.
- Pour lemon juice and olive oil on top of chicken.
- Bake chicken in preheated oven for 35-40 minutes.

- Serve and enjoy.

Per Serving: Net Carbs: 2.6g; Calories: 560; Total Fat: 31.6g; Saturated Fat: 11.8g Protein: 63.1g; Carbs: 2.9g; Fiber: 0.3g; Sugar: 0.4g; Fat 52% Protein 46% Carbs 2%

DAY-17 BREAKFAST

Bacon Avocado Quiche

Serves: 6 Preparation time: 10 minutes Cooking time: 30 minutes

6 eggs
1 avocado, peeled and chopped
½ cup bacon, cooked and crumbled
½ cup mozzarella cheese
¼ cup coconut milk
¼ tsp black pepper
¼ tsp salt

- Preheat the oven to 176 C 350 F.
- Spray pie dish with cooking spray and set aside.

- In a large bowl, whisk together eggs, coconut milk, pepper and salt until well combined.
- Add avocado, bacon and cheese and stir well.
- Pour egg mixture into the prepared pie dish and bake in preheated oven for 30 minutes.
- Serve and enjoy.

Per Serving: Net Carbs: 1.5g; Calories: 255 Total Fat: 20.4g; Saturated Fat: 6.2g Protein: 14.7g; Carbs: 3.8g; Fiber: 2.3g; Sugar: 0.6g; Fat 73% Protein 24% Carbs 3%

DAY-17 LUNCH

Perfect Geek Salad

Serves: 6 Preparation time: 10 minutes Cooking time: 5 minutes

2 cucumbers, peeled and chopped
2 tbsp olive oil
2 tbsp fresh dill, chopped
4 oz feta cheese, cubed
2 cups grape tomatoes, halved
Pepper
Salt

- Add all ingredients into the mixing bowl and toss well to combine.
- Serve and enjoy.

Per Serving: Net Carbs: 5.9g; Calories: 118; Total Fat: 9g; Saturated Fat: 3.6g Protein: 4.1g; Carbs: 7.3g; Fiber: 1.4g; Sugar: 4g; Fat 67% Protein 13% Carbs 20%

DAY-17 DINNER

Zucchini Cheese Casserole

Serves: 6 Preparation time: 10 minutes Cooking time: 25 minutes

4 cup zucchini, grated
12 cup parmesan cheese, grated
2 eggs
1 tbsp garlic, minced
12 cup onion, diced
12 cup cheddar cheese, shredded
1 cup mozzarella cheese, shredded
12 tsp salt

- Preheat the oven to 375 F.
- Spray baking dish with cooking spray and set aside.
- Add zucchini and salt into the colander and set aside for 10 minutes.
- Squeeze out all liquid from zucchini.
- In a large mixing bowl, combine together zucchini, cheddar cheese, mozzarella cheese, 12 parmesan

cheese, eggs, garlic, and onion and pour into the prepared baking dish.
- Bake in preheated oven for 25 minutes.
- Serve and enjoy.

Per Serving: Net Carbs: 3.2g; Calories: 140; Total Fat: 8.6g; Saturated Fat: 5g Protein: 10.7g; Carbs: 4.3g; Fiber: 1.1g; Sugar: 1.9g; Fat 58% Protein 32% Carbs 10%

DAY-18 BREAKFAST

Healthy Spinach Quiche

Serves: 6 Preparation time: 15 minutes Cooking time: 40 minutes

6 eggs
1 tsp lemon zest
Pinch of nutmeg
8 oz cheddar cheese, grated
¾ cup heavy cream
2 oz onion, sliced
16 oz frozen spinach, thawed and squeezed
13 lb bacon, cooked and chopped

¼ tsp pepper

¾ tsp salt

- Spray 8*8 pie dish with cooking spray and set aside.
- Preheat the oven to 176 C 350 F.
- In a large mixing bowl, add all ingredients and mix using electric mixer until well combined.
- Pour quiche mixture into the prepared pie dish and bake in preheated oven for 40 minutes.
- Serve and enjoy.

Per Serving: Net Carbs: 3.5g; Calories: 425 Total Fat: 33.3g; Saturated Fat: 16.3g Protein: 26.9g; Carbs: 5.4g; Fiber: 1.9g; Sugar: 1.3g; Fat 70% Protein 26% Carbs 4%

DAY-18 LUNCH

Healthy Mediterranean Salad

Serves: 6   Preparation time: 10 minutes   Cooking time: 10 minutes

½ cup feta cheese, crumbled

13 cup onion, sliced

1 cup artichoke hearts, chopped

2 cups cucumber, chopped

2 cups grape tomatoes, halved
For dressing:
1 garlic clove, minced
4 tsp apple cider vinegar
2 tbsp sun-dried tomatoes
6 tbsp olive oil
18 tsp black pepper
¼ tsp sea salt

- Add olive oil, garlic, vinegar, sun-dried tomatoes, pepper, and salt into the blender and blend until smooth.
- In a large mixing bowl, mix together feta cheese, onion, artichoke hearts, cucumber, and grape tomatoes.
- Pour dressing over salad and toss well to combine.
- Serve and enjoy.

Per Serving: Net Carbs: 5.3g; Calories: 186; Total Fat: 16.9g; Saturated Fat: 3.9g Protein: 3.5g; Carbs: 7.7g; Fiber: 2.4g; Sugar: 3.6g; Fat 81% Protein 7% Carbs 12%

DAY-18 DINNER

Tasty Pumpkin Spiced Soup

Serves: 4 Preparation time: 10 minutes Cooking time: 45 minutes

1 cup pumpkin puree
4 tbsp butter
1 1⁄2 cups vegetable broth
1⁄2 cup heavy cream
1 bay leaf
1⁄8 tsp nutmeg
1⁄4 tsp coriander
1⁄2 tsp ginger, minced
2 garlic cloves, minced
1⁄4 onion, chopped
1⁄4 tsp cinnamon
1⁄2 tsp pepper
1⁄2 tsp salt

- Melt butter in a saucepan over medium-low heat.
- Add ginger, garlic, and onion to the pan and sauté for 2-3 minutes.
- Add spices and stir well and cook for 2 minutes.
- Add broth and pumpkin puree and stir well.

- Bring to boil then reduce heat to low and simmer for 20 minutes.
- Puree the soup using immersion blender until smooth then simmer for another 20 minutes.
- Remove pan from heat and add heavy cream and stir well.
- Serve and enjoy.

Per Serving: Net Carbs: 5.2g; Calories: 196; Total Fat: 17.8g; Saturated Fat: 11g Protein: 3.2g; Carbs: 7.3g; Fiber: 2.1 g; Sugar: 2.7g; Fat 83% Protein 7% Carbs 10%

DAY-19 BREAKFAST

Almond Pumpkin Pancake

Serves: 4 Preparation time: 10 minutes Cooking time: 10 minutes

4 eggs
2 tbsp butter
2 tsp liquid stevia
1 tsp baking powder
½ tsp cinnamon
½ cup pumpkin puree
1 cup almond flour

- In a bowl, whisk together almond flour, stevia, baking powder, cinnamon, pumpkin puree, and eggs until well combined.
- Melt ½ tablespoon of butter in a pan over medium heat.
- Pour a heaping spoonful pancake batter into the melted butter and make round pancake.
- Cook pancake until lightly browned from both the sides.
- Serve and enjoy.

Per Serving: Net Carbs: 3.3g; Calories: 166 Total Fat: 13.7g; Saturated Fat: 5.3g Protein: 7.5g; Carbs: 5.1g; Fiber: 1.8g; Sugar: 1.6g; Fat 74% Protein 18% Carbs 8%

DAY-19 LUNCH

Refreshing Creamy Cucumber Salad

Serves: 6 Preparation time: 10 minutes Cooking time: 5 minutes

3 cucumbers, peeled and sliced
2 tbsp fresh chives, chopped
2 tbsp mayonnaise
½ cup sour cream
1 small onion, sliced
Pepper
Salt

- Add all ingredients into the large mixing bowl and mix well to combine.
- Place in refrigerator for 30 minutes.
- Serve chilled and enjoy.

Per Serving: Net Carbs: 6.2g; Calories: 69; Total Fat: 4.4g; Saturated Fat: 1.1g Protein: 1.4g; Carbs: 7.2g; Fiber: 1g; Sugar: 3g; Fat 57% Protein 8% Carbs 35%

DAY-19 DINNER

Herb Chicken

Serves: 10 Preparation time: 10 minutes Cooking time: 4 hours

6 chicken breasts, skinless and boneless

12 tsp thyme

1 tsp dried oregano

4 garlic cloves

1 medium onion, sliced

14 oz can tomatoes, diced

1 tsp dried basil

1 tsp dried rosemary

1 tbsp olive oil

12 cup balsamic vinegar

Pepper

Salt

- Add all ingredients into the slow cooker and stir well.
- Cover slow cooker with lid and cook on high for 4 hours.

- Stir well and serve.

Per Serving: Net Carbs: 2.7g; Calories: 197; Total Fat: 8g; Saturated Fat: 2g Protein: 25.9g; Carbs: 3.8g; Fiber: 1.1g; Sugar: 1.9g; Fat 39% Protein 55% Carbs 6%

DAY-20 BREAKFAST

Blueberry Almond Coconut Flour Casserole

Serves: 12 Preparation time: 10 minutes Cooking time: 25 minutes

3 eggs
1 cup blueberries
½ tsp vanilla
1 ¼ cup coconut milk
8 drops liquid stevia
½ tsp baking soda
1 ½ tsp baking powder
¼ cup coconut flour
1 12 cup almond flour
½ tsp salt

- Preheat the oven to 190 C 375 F.
- Spray 9*13 baking dish with cooking spray and set aside.
- In a large bowl, whisk together almond flour, baking soda, baking powder, coconut flour, and salt.
- Make in the center of almond flour mixture. Add eggs, coconut milk, vanilla, and stevia. Mix until well combined.
- Add blueberries and fold well.
- Pour into the prepared baking dish and bake in preheated oven for 20-25 minutes.
- Serve and enjoy.

Per Serving: Net Carbs: 3.5g; Calories: 111 Total Fat: 9.2g; Saturated Fat: 6.1g Protein: 3.1g; Carbs: 5.6g; Fiber: 2.1g; Sugar: 2.4g; Fat 75% Protein 12% Carbs 13%

DAY-20 LUNCH

Delicious Zucchini Soup

Serves: 4 Preparation time: 10 minutes Cooking time: 20 minutes

3 medium zucchini, chopped
2 tbsp sour cream
32 oz chicken broth
2 garlic cloves
½ small onion, quartered
Pepper
Salt

- Add broth, zucchini, garlic, and onion to the saucepan and heat over medium heat. Bring to boil.
- Turn heat to low and simmer for 20 minutes.
- Puree the soup using immersion blender until smooth and creamy.
- Add sour cream and stir well.
- Season soup with pepper and salt.
- Serve hot and enjoy.

Per Serving: Net Carbs: 5.5g; Calories: 78; Total Fat: 2.8g; Saturated Fat: 1.2g Protein: 6.8g; Carbs: 7.4g; Fiber: 1.9g; Sugar: 3.6g; Fat 35% Protein 35% Carbs 30%

DAY-20 DINNER

Zucchini Cheese Gratin

Serves: 9 Preparation time: 10 minutes Cooking time: 50 minutes

4 cups raw zucchini, sliced
12 cup heavy whipping cream
1 12 cups pepper jack cheese, shredded
1 onion, sliced
12 tsp garlic powder
2 tbsp butter
Pepper
Salt

- Preheat the oven to 190 C 375 F.
- Spray oven safe pan with cooking spray.
- Add 13 sliced onion and zucchini in pan and season with pepper and salt.
- Sprinkle 12 cup cheese over sliced onion and zucchini.
- In a microwave safe dish, combine together heavy whipping cream, butter, and garlic powder.

- Microwave for 1 minute or until butter is melted.
- Pour heavy cream mixture over sliced zucchini and onion.
- Bake in preheated oven for 45 minutes.
- Serve and enjoy.

Per Serving: Net Carbs: 3g; Calories: 126; Total Fat: 10.5g; Saturated Fat: 6.5g Protein: 4.9g; Carbs: 3.8g; Fiber: 0.8g; Sugar: 1.4g; Fat 75% Protein 15% Carbs 10%

DAY-21 BREAKFAST

Creamy Egg Scrambled

Serves: 3 Preparation time: 10 minutes Cooking time: 15 minutes

5 eggs
3 oz cream cheese
13 cup whipping cream
¼ cup onion, chopped
2 tbsp butter
1 tbsp parsley, chopped
Pepper

Salt

- Melt butter in a large pan over low heat.
- Add onion to the pan and sauté until softened.
- Add cream cheese and cream and stir until cream cheese melted.
- In a bowl, whisk eggs with pepper and salt.
- Pour egg mixture into the pan and stir until eggs are set.
- Garnish with parsley and serve.

Per Serving: Net Carbs: 2.4g; Calories: 315 Total Fat: 29g; Saturated Fat: 15.9g Protein: 11.9g; Carbs: 2.7g; Fiber: 0.3g; Sugar: 1.1g; Fat 82% Protein 15% Carbs 3%

DAY-21 LUNCH

Easy Chicken Fajitas

Serves: 6 Preparation time: 10 minutes Cooking time: 10 minutes

4 chicken breasts, skinless and boneless
12 cup onion, sliced
12 cup bell pepper, sliced
12 cup water
1 packet fajita seasoning

- Add all ingredients into the instant pot and stir well.
- Seal pot with lid and cook on high pressure for 10 minutes.
- Release pressure using quick release method than open the lid.
- Shred the chicken using fork.
- Serve and enjoy.

Per Serving: Net Carbs: 1.4g; Calories: 192; Total Fat: 7.2g; Saturated Fat: 2g

Protein: 28.4g; Carbs: 1.7g; Fiber: 0.3g; Sugar: 0.9g; Fat 35% Protein 61% Carbs 4%

DAY-21 DINNER

Zucchini Noodles

Serves: 2 Preparation time: 10 minutes Cooking time: 10 minutes

1 zucchini, spiralized into noodles
1 tbsp butter
12 cup water
23 cup cheddar cheese, shredded
2 tbsp almond milk
1 tsp salt

- Add noodles, salt, and water in a saucepan and bring to boil.
- Boil noodles until soft and water are completely absorbed.
- Reduce heat to low and add cheese, almond milk, and butter. Stir well to combine.
- Serve and enjoy.

Per Serving: Net Carbs: 3.2g; Calories: 253; Total Fat: 22g; Saturated Fat: 14.8g Protein: 11g; Carbs: 4.6g; Fiber: 1.4g; Sugar: 2.4g; Fat 78% Protein 17% Carbs 5%

DAY-22 BREAKFAST

Cauliflower Cheese Bread

Serves: 10 Preparation time: 10 minutes Cooking time: 45 minutes

1 medium cauliflower head, grated

1 tsp basil

1 cup cheddar cheese, divided

2 large eggs

34 cup yogurt

12 cup parmesan cheese

1 tbsp rosemary

12 tsp thyme

1 tsp oregano

14 tsp pepper

12 tsp salt

- Preheat the oven to 204 C 400 F.
- Add all ingredients into the mixing bowl and mix until well combined.
- Pour batter on cookie sheet and line with parchment paper until evenly spread.
- Bake in preheated oven for 40-45 minutes.
- Cut bread into the pieces and serve.

Per Serving: Net Carbs: 3.4g; Calories: 106 Total Fat: 6.2g; Saturated Fat: 3.6g Protein: 7.8g; Carbs: 5.1g; Fiber: 1.7g; Sugar: 2.8g; Fat 55% Protein 31% Carbs 14%

DAY-22 LUNCH

Mayo Cabbage Coleslaw

Serves: 4 Preparation time: 10 minutes Cooking time: 30 minutes

3 cups cabbage, shredded
1 tsp dried dill
1 tbsp red wine vinegar
13 cup mayonnaise
5 drops liquid stevia
12 tsp onion powder
1 tsp salt

- In a large bowl, mix together mayonnaise, stevia, onion powder, dill, vinegar, and salt.
- Add shredded cabbage to the bowl and stir well to combine. Place in refrigerator for 30 minutes.
- Serve and enjoy.

Per Serving: Net Carbs: 2.1g; Calories: 136; Total Fat: 13.4g;   Saturated   Fat: 2g

Protein: 0.8g; Carbs: 3.5g; Fiber: 1.4g; Sugar: 1.8g; Fat 90% Protein 3% Carbs 7%

DAY-22 DINNER

Cauliflower Cheese Gratin

Serves: 4 Preparation time: 10 minutes Cooking time: 25 minutes

4 cups cauliflower florets
13 cup heavy whipping cream
4 tbsp butter
6 pepper jack cheese slices
Pepper
Salt

- Add cauliflower florets, pepper, salt, heavy whipping cream and butter in oven safe dish.
- Place dish in oven and microwave for 25 minutes.
- Slightly mash the cauliflower florets using back of spoon.
- Place cheese slices over cauliflower mixture and microwave for 2 minutes or until cheese melted.
- Serve and enjoy.

Per Serving: Net Carbs: 3.1g; Calories: 281; Total Fat: 24.3g; Saturated Fat: 14.9g Protein: 9.8g; Carbs: 5.6g; Fiber: 2.5g; Sugar: 2.4g; Fat 79% Protein 15% Carbs 6%

DAY-23 BREAKFAST

Herb Cauliflower Bread

Serves: 10 Preparation time: 10 minutes Cooking time: 30 minutes

2 eggs

14 tsp red chili flakes, crushed

2 tsp fresh parsley, chopped

12 cup parmesan cheese, grated

12 tsp oregano, dried

2 garlic cloves, minced

1 large cauliflower head, grated

3 cups mozzarella cheese, shredded and divided

14 tsp pepper

12 tsp salt

- Preheat the oven to 218 C 425 F.
- Line baking tray with parchment paper.

- In a mixing bowl, combine together cauliflower, 1 cup mozzarella cheese, oregano, garlic, parmesan cheese, eggs, pepper, and salt.
- Place dough on baking tray and pat into a crust.
- Bake in preheated oven for 25 minutes.
- Sprinkle remaining cheese, parsley, and red chili flakes and bake for 5 minutes more or until cheese are melted.
- Cut into slices and serve.

Per Serving: Net Carbs: 2.9g; Calories: 89 Total Fat: 4.3g; Saturated Fat: 2.4g Protein: 7.6g; Carbs: 5.1g; Fiber: 2.2g; Sugar: 2.1g; Fat 47% Protein 37% Carbs 16%

DAY-23 LUNCH

Cabbage Dill Cucumber Salad

Serves: 8 Preparation time: 10 minutes Cooking time: 10 minutes

12 head cabbage, shredded
2 tbsp green onions, chopped
2 tbsp fresh dill, chopped
2 cucumbers, sliced
3 tbsp olive oil
12 lemon juice
Pepper
Salt

- Add shredded cabbage and 1 tsp salt into the bowl and set aside to release juices.
- Add remaining ingredients to the cabbage bowl and stir well.
- Serve and enjoy.

Per Serving: Net Carbs: 4.2g; Calories: 71; Total Fat: 5.4g; Saturated Fat: 0.8g

Protein: 1.3g; Carbs: 5.9g; Fiber: 1.7g; Sugar: 2.8g; Fat 69% Protein 8% Carbs 23%

DAY-23 DINNER

Cheese Cauliflower Rice

Serves: 6 Preparation time: 10 minutes Cooking time: 5 minutes

1 cauliflower head, cut into florets
14 tsp garlic powder
2 oz cream cheese
2.5 oz cheddar cheese, shredded
14 tsp pepper
14 tsp salt

- Add cauliflower florets into the food processor and process until it looks like rice.
- Transfer cauliflower rice to the baking dish and microwave for 5 minutes.
- Add cream cheese and cheddar cheese and stir until melted.
- Add garlic powder, pepper, and salt and stir well.
- Serve and enjoy.

Per Serving: Net Carbs: 1.8g; Calories: 92; Total Fat: 7.3g; Saturated Fat: 4.6g Protein: 4.6g; Carbs: 2.9g; Fiber: 1.1g; Sugar: 1.2g; Fat 72% Protein 20% Carbs 8%

DAY-24 BREAKFAST

Vanilla protein Muffins

Serves: 6   Preparation time: 5 minutes   Cooking time: 25 minutes

4 eggs

1 scoop whey protein powder

1 tsp vanilla

2 tbsp butter

4 oz cream cheese

- Spray muffin tray with cooking spray and set aside.
- In a bowl, melt cream cheese and butter.
- Add eggs, vanilla, and whey protein in a bowl and mix until well combined.
- Pour batter into the prepared muffin tray and bake at 176 C 350 F for 25 minutes.
- Serve and enjoy.

Per Serving: Net Carbs: 1.4g; Calories: 164 Total Fat: 13.7g; Saturated Fat: 7.6g Protein: 8.9g; Carbs: 1.4g; Fiber: 0g; Sugar: 0.5g; Fat 75% Protein 21% Carbs 4%

DAY-24 LUNCH

Healthy Coconut Spinach Soup

Serves: 4 Preparation time: 105 minutes Cooking time: 15 minutes

2 cups baby spinach, wash and pat dry
2 cups vegetable broth
12 tsp ginger, grated
12 onion, diced
2 cups cauliflower florets
1 tbsp olive oil
1 tbsp coconut cream
1 cup fresh parsley, chopped

- Heat olive oil in a saucepan over medium heat.
- Add onion and sauté until translucent. Add cauliflower and cook until softened.
- Add broth and stir well. Cover saucepan and bring to boil.
- Once vegetable is soften than add spinach, coconut cream, ginger, and parsley. Stir until spinach wilted.

- Remove from heat and puree the soup using immersion blender until smooth.
- Serve and enjoy.

Per Serving: Net Carbs: 3.8g; Calories: 85; Total Fat: 5.3g; Saturated Fat: 1.5g Protein: 4.6g; Carbs: 6.3g; Fiber: 2.5g; Sugar: 2.5g; Fat 58% Protein 23% Carbs 19%

DAY-24 DINNER

Baked Broccoli

Serves: 4 Preparation time: 10 minutes Cooking time: 10 minutes

1 broccoli stalk, cut into florets
14 cup parmesan cheese, grated
12 cup heavy cream
2 garlic cloves, minced
12 cup gruyere, shredded
12 cup mozzarella cheese, shredded
1 tbsp butter
Pepper
Salt

- Preheat the oven to 190 C 375 F.
- Melt butter in an oven-safe pan over medium-high heat.
- Add broccoli florets in a pan and season with pepper and salt.
- Cook broccoli florets for 5 minutes or until tender. Add garlic and stir for 1 minute.

- Add heavy cream on top of broccoli then top with parmesan, gruyere, and mozzarella cheese.
- Place pan in preheated oven and bake broccoli for 10 minutes.
- Serve and enjoy.

Per Serving: Net Carbs: 2g; Calories: 303; Total Fat: 22.5g; Saturated Fat: 14.2g Protein: 18.3g; Carbs: 2.6g; Fiber: 0.6g; Sugar: 0.5g; Fat 69% Protein 26% Carbs 5%

DAY-25 BREAKFAST

Coconut Kale Muffins

Serves: 8 Preparation time: 10 minutes Cooking time: 30 minutes

6 eggs

12 cup coconut milk

1 cup kale, chopped

14 cup chives, chopped

Pepper

Salt

- Preheat the oven to 176 C 350 F.
- Spray muffin tray with cooking spray and set aside.
- Add all ingredients into the bowl and whisk well to combined.
- Pour mixture into the prepared muffin tray and bake in preheated oven for 30 minutes.
- Serve and enjoy.

Per Serving: Net Carbs: 1.5g; Calories: 86 Total Fat: 6.9g; Saturated Fat: 4.2g Protein: 4.8g; Carbs: 2g; Fiber: 0.5g; Sugar: 0.8g; Fat 72% Protein 22% Carbs 6%

DAY-25 LUNCH

Garlic Herb Baked Mushrooms

Serves: 6 Preparation time: 10 minutes Cooking time: 20 minutes

1 lb button mushrooms, scrubbed and stems trimmed
2 tbsp olive oil
4 tbsp balsamic vinegar
14 tsp black pepper
12 tsp dried basil
12 tsp dried oregano
3 garlic cloves, crushed
1 tsp sea salt

- Preheat the oven to 215 C 425 F.
- Spray a baking tray with cooking spray and set aside.
- In a mixing bowl, mix together vinegar, basil, oregano, garlic, olive oil, pepper, and salt.
- Stir in mushrooms and let sit for 15 minutes.
- Spread mushrooms onto the prepared baking tray and bake in preheated oven for 15-20 minutes.

- Serve and enjoy.

Per Serving: Net Carbs: 2.3g; Calories: 61; Total Fat: 4.9g; Saturated Fat: 0.7g Protein: 2.5g; Carbs: 3.2g; Fiber: 0.9g; Sugar: 1.4g; Fat 71% Protein 14% Carbs 15%

DAY-25 DINNER

Parmesan Spinach Pie

Serves: 6 Preparation time: 10 minutes Cooking time: 60 minutes

4 eggs
12 cup heavy cream
16 oz cottage cheese
2 tbsp parmesan cheese, grated
1 tsp garlic, minced
8 oz mushrooms, sliced
10 oz fresh spinach
12 cup mozzarella cheese, shredded
14 tsp nutmeg
12 tsp pepper
2 tsp olive oil
1 tsp salt

- Preheat the oven to 176 C 350 F.
- Heat oil in a pan over medium heat.

- Add mushrooms and garlic in a pan and sauté until tender.
- Add spinach, nutmeg, pepper, and salt and cook until spinach is wilted.
- Drain spinach and mushrooms mixture.
- Sprinkle parmesan cheese into the 9" pie dish.
- In a bowl, whisk together eggs, cottage cheese, and cream and stir well.
- Add mushroom and spinach mixture and stir well.
- Pour mushroom and spinach mixture into a pie dish and bake in preheated oven for 50 minutes.
- Slice and serve.

Per Serving: Net Carbs: 5.1g; Calories: 198; Total Fat: 11.1g; Saturated Fat: 5.2g Protein: 18.6g; Carbs: 6.6g; Fiber: 1.5g; Sugar: 1.4g; Fat 51% Protein 38% Carbs 11%

DAY-26 BREAKFAST

Spicy & Creamy Egg Scrambled

Serves: 2 Preparation time: 10 minutes Cooking time: 10 minutes

4 eggs

2 tbsp cilantro, chopped

13 cup heavy cream

1 tomato, diced

1 Serrano chili pepper, chopped

2 tbsp scallions, sliced

14 tsp black pepper

3 tbsp butter

12 tsp salt

- Melt butter in a pan over medium heat.
- Add tomato and chili pepper and sauté for 2 minutes.
- In a bowl, whisk together eggs, cilantro, cream, pepper, and salt.
- Pour egg mixture into the pan and stir until egg is set.
- Top with scallions and serve.

Per Serving: Net Carbs: 3g; Calories: 358 Total Fat: 33.5g; Saturated Fat: 18.3g Protein: 12.1g; Carbs: 3.6g; Fiber: 0.6g; Sugar: 1.7g; Fat 84% Protein 13% Carbs 3%

DAY-26 LUNCH

Creamy Cauliflower Broccoli Mashed

Serves: 4 Preparation time: 10 minutes Cooking time: 10 minutes

2 cups cauliflower florets
1 tbsp olive oil
2 cups broccoli florets
3 garlic cloves, peeled
12 tsp pepper
12 tsp salt

- Heat olive oil in a pan over medium heat.
- Add cauliflower, broccoli, and salt in a pan and sauté until softened.
- Transfer vegetables and garlic to the food processor and process until smooth.
- Season with pepper and salt.
- Serve and enjoy.

Per Serving: Net Carbs: 4g; Calories: 62; Total Fat: 3.7g; Saturated Fat: 0.5g

Protein: 2.4g; Carbs: 6.6g; Fiber: 2.6g; Sugar: 2g; Fat 56% Protein 17% Carbs 27%

DAY-26 DINNER

Almond Jalapeno Pizza

Serves: 4 Preparation time: 10 minutes Cooking time: 20 minutes

13 cup almond flour

14 tsp garlic powder

1 egg, beaten

34 cup mozzarella cheese, shredded

1 cup cheddar cheese, shredded

2 jalapeno pepper, sliced

2 oz cream cheese

- Preheat the oven to 176 C 350 F.
- In a small bowl, add mozzarella cheese and cream cheese. Microwave on high for 20 seconds or until melted.
- Add remaining ingredients to the melted cheese and stir well.
- Spray 10" pan with cooking spray and spread the dough out evenly.
- Bake in preheated oven for 10 minutes.

- Top with jalapenos and cheese and cook for 10 minutes more.
- Serve and enjoy.

Per Serving: Net Carbs: 1.6g; Calories: 210; Total Fat: 17.5g; Saturated Fat: 10.1g Protein: 11.6g; Carbs: 2.1g; Fiber: 0.5g; Sugar: 0.6g; Fat 75% Protein 22% Carbs 3%

DAY-27 BREAKFAST

Cinnamon Cream Egg Scrambled

Serves: 2   Preparation time: 5 minutes   Cooking time: 10 minutes

4 eggs
14 tsp ground cinnamon
2 tbsp cream
1 tbsp butter

- In a bowl, whisk together cream and eggs until smooth.
- Melt butter in a pan over medium heat.
- Add egg mixture in a pan and cook until egg is set.

- Top with cinnamon and serve.

Per Serving: Net Carbs: 1.1g; Calories: 185 Total Fat: 15.2g; Saturated Fat: 6.8g Protein: 11.2g; Carbs: 1.3g; Fiber: 0.2g; Sugar: 0.9g; Fat 73% Protein 24% Carbs 3%

DAY-27 LUNCH

Paprika Egg Cucumber Salad

Serves: 4 Preparation time: 10 minutes Cooking time: 5 minutes

6 hard-boiled eggs

1 avocado, peel and cubed

1 medium cucumber, peeled and chopped

12 tsp paprika

14 cup mayonnaise

- Peel the eggs and cut into pieces.
- Add all ingredients into the mixing bowl and toss well to combined.
- Serve and enjoy.

Per Serving: Net Carbs: 2.9g; Calories: 211; Total Fat: 17.9g; Saturated Fat: 3.8g

Protein: 9.1g; Carbs: 4.1g; Fiber: 1.2g; Sugar: 1.8g; Fat 76% Protein 18% Carbs 6%

DAY-27 DINNER

Spinach Casserole

Serves: 6 Preparation time: 10 minutes Cooking time: 35 minutes

2 eggs

1 14 cup cheddar cheese, shredded

12 red pepper, chopped

2 cups frozen spinach, thawed and drained

1 12 cups egg whites

12 green pepper, chopped

12 onion, chopped

1 cup mushrooms, sliced

Pepper

Salt

- Preheat the oven to 176 C 375 F.
- Spray casserole dish with cooking spray and set aside.
- Heat pan over medium-high heat.
- Add chopped vegetables except spinach to the pan and sauté for few minutes until vegetables are soft.

- Add vegetables to the bottom of casserole dish and spread the vegetables to the dish.
- Add spinach to the vegetables and spread well.
- Whisk eggs and egg whites in a small bowl and season with pepper and salt.
- Pour egg mixture over the vegetables.
- Sprinkle with shredded cheese.
- Bake in preheated oven for 35 minutes.
- Serve and enjoy.

Per Serving: Net Carbs: 2.8g; Calories: 161; Total Fat: 9.5g; Saturated Fat: 5.4g Protein: 15.3g; Carbs: 3.7g; Fiber: 0.9g; Sugar: 2g; Fat 54% Protein 39% Carbs 7%

DAY-28 BREAKFAST

Flavorful Cheese Quiche

Serves: 8   Preparation time: 5 minutes   Cooking time: 45 minutes

12 eggs
8 oz cheddar cheese, grated
34 cup butter

4 oz cream cheese, softened

Pepper

Salt

- Add half cup cheese to the 10-inch pie pan.
- Add eggs, cream cheese, and butter into the blender and blend until well combined.
- Pour egg mixture over cheese in pie pan. Season with pepper and salt.
- Sprinkle remaining cheese on top of egg mixture and bake at 162 C 325 F for 45 minutes.
- Serve and enjoy.

Per Serving: Net Carbs: 1.3g; Calories: 411 Total Fat: 38.2g; Saturated Fat: 22.1g Protein: 16.6g; Carbs: 1.3g; Fiber: 0g; Sugar: 0.7g; Fat 83% Protein 16% Carbs 1%

DAY-28 LUNCH

Easy Caesar Salad

Serves: 8 Preparation time: 10 minutes Cooking time: 5 minutes

8 cups romaine lettuce, chopped
2 tbsp fresh lemon juice
14 cup olive oil
14 cup parmesan cheese, grated
14 tsp garlic powder
1 tbsp mayonnaise
14 tsp pepper
18 tsp salt

- In a large bowl, combine together olive oil, garlic powder, mayonnaise, and lemon juice.
- Add lettuce and cheese in a bowl. Season with pepper and salt.
- Cover bowl and place in refrigerator for 1 hour.
- Toss well and serve.

Per Serving: Net Carbs: 1.9g; Calories: 145; Total Fat: 11.5g; Saturated Fat: 4g

Protein: 6.3g; Carbs: 2.3g; Fiber: 0.4g; Sugar: 0.8g; Fat 74% Protein 19% Carbs 7%

DAY-28 DINNER

Cheese Chicken Casserole

Serves: 8 Preparation time: 10 minutes Cooking time: 40 minutes

2 lbs cooked chicken, shredded

6 oz cream cheese, softened

4 oz butter, melted

6 oz ham, cut into small pieces

5 oz Swiss cheese

1 oz fresh lemon juice

1 tbsp Dijon mustard

½ tsp salt

- Preheat the oven to 176 C 350 F.
- Place chicken in the bottom of baking dish then layer ham pieces on top.
- Add butter, lemon juice, mustard, cream cheese, and salt into the blender and blend until a thick sauce.
- Spread sauce over top of chicken and ham mixture in the baking dish.

- Arrange Swiss cheese slices on top of sauce.
- Bake in preheated oven for 40 minutes.
- Serve and enjoy.

Per Serving: Net Carbs: 2.1g; Calories: 451; Total Fat: 29.2g; Saturated Fat: 16.7g Protein: 43g; Carbs: 2.5g; Fiber: 0.4g; Sugar: 0.4g; Fat 59% Protein 39% Carbs 2%

DAY-29 BREAKFAST

Tasty Cauliflower Frittata

Serves: 1 Preparation time: 10 minutes Cooking time: 15 minutes

1 egg
12 tbsp onion, diced
5 tbsp cauliflower rice
1 tbsp olive oil
14 tsp turmeric
18 tsp black pepper
Salt

- Add all ingredients except oil into the bowl and mix well to combine.
- Heat oil in a pan over medium heat.
- Using spoon scoop the mixture and pour into the hot pan and cook for 3-4 minutes or until lightly golden brown.
- Serve and enjoy.

Per Serving: Net Carbs: 1.9g; Calories: 195 Total Fat: 18.5g; Saturated Fat: 3.4g Protein: 6.3g; Carbs: 3g; Fiber: 1.1g; Sugar: 1.3g; Fat 85% Protein 12% Carbs 3%

DAY-29 LUNCH

Flavors Squash Soup

Serves: 8 Preparation time: 10 minutes Cooking time: 35 minutes

1 lb butternut squash, peeled and diced
5 tbsp olive oil, divided
12 cup heavy cream
1 bay leaf
4 cups vegetable broth
3 garlic cloves, minced
1 tsp sea salt

- Heat 1 tablespoon of olive oil in a saucepan over medium heat.
- Add butternut squash, salt, and garlic and sauté until lightly golden brown.
- Add broth, remaining oil, and bay leaves in a saucepan. Bring to boil.
- Simmer for 30 minutes or until squash cooked completely.
- Discard bay leaves from soup.

- Puree the soup using immersion blender until smooth and creamy.
- Add heavy cream and stir well.
- Serve and enjoy.

Per Serving: Net Carbs: 6.3g; Calories: 171; Total Fat: 14.5g; Saturated Fat: 5g Protein: 3.1g; Carbs: 7.5g; Fiber: 1.2g; Sugar: 1.6g; Fat 77% Protein 8% Carbs 15%

DAY-29 DINNER

Spicy Chicken Curry

Serves: 6 Preparation time: 10 minutes Cooking time: 20 minutes

1 ½ lbs chicken thighs, skinless, boneless, and cut into pieces
1 cup tomatoes, chopped
1 tbsp jalapeno pepper, minced
2 tbsp ginger, diced
2 tbsp olive oil
¼ cup fresh cilantro, chopped
2 tbsp fresh lemon juice

2 tsp cayenne

1 tsp garam masala

2 tsp turmeric

- Heat olive oil in a pan over medium heat.
- Add jalapenos and ginger to the pan and sauté for 2-3 minutes.
- Add chicken and sear chicken from both the sides. Add tomatoes and stir well.
- Add all spices and stir well and cook until chicken is completely cooked and tomatoes soften.
- Add lemon juice and stir well.
- Garnish with chopped cilantro and serve.

Per Serving: Net Carbs: 2.4g; Calories: 273; Total Fat: 13.5g; Saturated Fat: 3.1g Protein: 33.4g; Carbs: 3.4g; Fiber: 1g; Sugar: 1.1g; Fat 46% Protein 50% Carbs 4%

DAY-30 BREAKFAST

Mushroom Asparagus Frittata

Serves: 4 Preparation time: 10 minutes Cooking time: 15 minutes

6 eggs

3 mushrooms, sliced

10 asparagus, chopped

14 cup half and half

2 tsp butter

1 cup mozzarella cheese, shredded

1 tsp black pepper

1 tsp salt

- Melt butter in oven safe pan over medium heat.
- Add mushrooms in a pan and sauté for 5 minutes.
- Add asparagus and sauté for 2 minutes.
- Meanwhile, in a bowl, whisk together eggs, half and half, pepper, and salt and pour over asparagus. Cook over medium heat until set.
- Sprinkle cheese on top and transfer pan to the oven and cook for 5 minutes.
- Cut into pieces and serve.

Per Serving: Net Carbs: 2.5g; Calories: 161 Total Fat: 11.6g; Saturated Fat: 5.1g Protein: 11.9g; Carbs: 3.4g; Fiber: 0.9g; Sugar: 1.3g; Fat 65% Protein 30% Carbs 5%

DAY-30 LUNCH

Simple Broccoli Omelet

Serves: 2 Preparation time: 10 minutes Cooking time: 10 minutes

4 eggs
1 tbsp olive oil
1 cup broccoli, chopped and cooked
1 tbsp fresh parsley, chopped
14 tsp pepper
12 tsp salt

- In a bowl, whisk eggs with pepper, and salt.
- Heat olive oil in a pan over medium heat.
- Add broccoli and eggs mixture into the pan and cook until set.
- Turn omelet to other side and cook until lightly golden brown.
- Garnish with chopped parsley.
- Serve and enjoy.

Per Serving: Net Carbs: 2.7g; Calories: 203; Total Fat: 15.9g; Saturated Fat: 3.7g

Protein: 12.4g; Carbs: 4g; Fiber: 1.3g; Sugar: 1.5g; Fat 71% Protein 25% Carbs 4%

DAY-30 DINNER

Meatloaf

Serves: 8 Preparation time: 10 minutes Cooking time: 40 minutes

2 eggs
12 cup parmesan cheese, grated
12 cup marinara sauce, sugar free
1 cup cottage cheese
1 lb mozzarella cheese, cut into cubes
2 lbs ground turkey
2 tsp Italian seasoning
14 cup basil pesto
1 tsp salt

- Preheat the oven to 204 C 400 F.
- Spray casserole dish with cooking spray and set aside.
- Add all ingredients into the mixing bowl and mix until well combined.
- Transfer bowl mixture to the prepared casserole dish and bake in preheated oven for 40 minutes.

- Serve and enjoy.

Per Serving: Net Carbs: 3.1g; Calories: 327; Total Fat: 17.7g; Saturated Fat: 4.8g Protein: 40.6g; Carbs: 3.5g; Fiber: 0.4g; Sugar: 1.7g; Fat 49% Protein 48% Carbs 3%

Part 2

Introduction

Meal preparation, also known as meal prep, is the process of planning and preparing of meals.

Meal prepping shouldn't be a hassle at all. Instead of making rushed trips to the grocery store and guessing about the numbers, there are simple rules that could come in handy for successful meal prep. For a majority of people, meal prep has shown that it is the secret to reaching their goals when it comes to being fit. As soon as you know how meal prep works, you will be amazed at the great results!

However, this process could be tedious to someone who is not used to it, and at times, it is even a hassle for the ones who have done it for a long time. Meal prep can take much of your time and if not done the right way, it can leave you discouraged and always rushing to the fast food joints. To be successful in meal prepping, you need to have a well laid out plan. This is important for you to have enough nutrients in your meals.

Tips for meal prepping
- **Plan ahead for your day**

Within the fitness circles, meal-prep Sunday is a well-respected day. This is because prepping on a Sunday does not affect your weekdays and is close enough to the beginning of the week. Prepping time will depend on the meals you are making. You can also prep the meals in two days if Sunday is not enough for you. Far from cutting down on the time you spend; splitting into two will also preserve the quality of your food.

- **Be sure of your numbers**

Before your start meal prepping, you need to know your number of meals and what those meals constitute.

Meals

Decide on the number of meals as well as the number of days that you will be preparing each. Other people find it convenient to prep only their lunch for each day because they can eat breakfast and dinner at home. For others, it is convenient for them to prep daily meals for the whole week, or even all the meals. Regardless of which path you choose, select an option that works best for you.

Macros

In case you are cycling carbs, you need to know your requirements for each day. Outline your daily macros with specific meal by meal requirements and place it somewhere in your kitchen. The refrigerator is the best place to stick your meal plan.

- *Use staple items*

It is always good to have diversity and variety within meals, but relying on exotic recipes will take much of your time. You should focus on foods that are easy to cook and store. I would recommend:

Protein
- Chicken breast
- Lean ground beef
- Pork tenderloin
- Flank steak
- Lean lunch meat(turkey breast, roast beef or ham and low fat beef jerky

Carbs
- Oats
- Quinoa
- Couscous
- Brown rice
- Wild rice
- Whole grain tortillas
- Bread

Healthy fats
- Almonds, walnuts

- Pecans
- Pistachios
- Pumpkin seeds
- Peanut butter
- Almond butter
- Olive oil
- Coconut oil

- **Shop for groceries**

Once you are sure of your numbers, ensure that you stock everything you require. This will help you save money and avoid wastage of food.

- **Buy a cooler or insulated meal bag**

It is always a good feeling to have a well-stocked fridge. If you only prep a meal a day, you can do without a fridge or meal bag. However, if they are more, you definitely need them.

There are a lot of good reasons for meal prepping but the main ones are saving time, money and healthy eating. This book will offer you sample recipes that will help you start out.

CHAPTER ONE

Recommended products for meal prep

- Rubbermaid set

- Slow cooker

- Griddler

- Rice cookerfood steamer

- Lunchbox set

- Ziploc storage bags

- Snack bags

- Dry erase markers

- Sharpies

Getting started

The basic steps for beginners are:
- Check your calendar so that you know how your schedule is.

- Take a look at your pantry and know what you have that you will need.

- Find out about some recipes.

- Make a list of groceries.

- After you shop, sort out the foods into the ones you will make immediately and later.

As soon as you get home from shopping:
- Wash and prepare your fruit and veggies. Cut them up, and store in containers in the fridge.

- Bake your chicken and brown your meat. You can shred or cube the chicken enough for you to use for the whole week. Additionally, you could split them into each container for a specific day.

- Cook your rice, pasta or anything else you need to and store in your containers.

- Do not forget to label each container; you can use sharpies on plastic bags and dry markers on plastic containers.

Meal prep for beginners

Everyone has heard this famous saying, "If you fail to prepare, you prepare to fail". This is mostly true when it comes to prepare your meals. A majority of people are always busy; be it a working mum or student, and it could be really difficult to cook all meals at home every day. This is where meal prep comes in.

Without meal prep, you are most likely to eat junk. Meal prep can have different meanings to various people, and so, it is advisable for you to find a routine that suits you well. Basically, meal prep is aimed at saving your time in the kitchen and making it simpler for you to eat healthy through the week. You may decide to prepare only breakfasts, dinners, snacks, or all the meals. In case you are always in a hurry in the mornings, preparing breakfast will greatly benefit you.

The first step in preparing meals is to invest in good quality containers. Also keep in mind that you will be warming your food, so select containers that are suitable for use in the microwave or oven.

The next step is the planning. It is vital to have a meal plan ready rather than going to shop for random things. For you to be successful in meal prep, you need to know what you will be cooking and when. Note down whatever you will be eating for breakfast, lunch, and dinner, break down the ingredients needed for the meals and how much you will need to last you for the period. It is also advisable to stick to tried and tested recipes. Furthermore, select recipes that can be prepared in advance and will not go bad fast.

After that, you can now start your preparation. Meal prep can be done in many ways but you need to select the method that suits your lifestyle. As for me, taste tops the list. Just like everybody else, I enjoy eating healthy foods with great taste. I always enjoy trying out new flavors such as spices, homemade marinades and toppings. Try and incorporate as much variety as you can possibly can, so that you will not get bored of eating the same thing on a daily basis.

When it comes to the time you spend on meal prep, you are the one to decide. You can even dedicate a whole day to meal prep, or spread it out. As for me, I find it convenient taking a few hours on Sunday night to do meal prep. The time I take usually depends on whatever am prepping. For instance, if there are meals or snacks that I enjoy while fresh, such as salad or veggies, then I just sort them in the same containers in the fridge and chop them up in the morning or just before I eat them. On the other hand, when I want more complex meals such as stir fries, I will chop all the veggies so that they are ready when it's time to cook.

Meal prep doesn't however mean that you have to pre-cook all your food. You can marinate your chicken breasts and place them in the freezer and when you are ready to use them, you just defrost. This also applies to homemade turkey burgers and many more similar dishes. Another tip is to make a large batch of your preferred sauces and refrigerate rather than making several smaller portions. If you enjoy your veggies freshly cooked, you can split them up for each meal and put them in containers so that they are ready to be steamed or cooked. Also, for meals that need a lot of chopping, it is better if you do that in advance. Fruit and nut portions can also be washed in advance so that they can be easily eaten on the go.

Sample recipes for meal prep

In case you are at home and in no hurry, you can poach eggs and toast your bread fresh. In case you want something more organized, you can pack each ingredient in a container and use them in the morning. This will save you time. You can chop mushrooms and set aside a portion of spinach in advance and cook them fresh on the day.

Cooked breakfast

- Two poached eggs.

- Two sliced dark rye bread, toasted.

- Two small mushrooms that are sliced and cooked.

- A small handful of cooked baby spinach.

- One regular coffee with a cup of low milk.

Snacks

You can portion out your berries and nut and seed mix and place in a container in the fridge.

- A cup, 100 grams of mixed berries

- 200g low fat yogurt

- 10g nut and seed mix

Lunch

If you wish to make this a few days in advance, you can put all the ingredients next to each other in the fridge or together in one container and prepare the following morning.

Tuna crispbreads

- Four rye crispbreads.

- 50g of drained tuna.

- Half of a small cucumber, sliced.

- 60g ricotta cheese, quarter cup.

Dinner

You can cook your chicken in advance.

Herb crusted chicken and chicken pea salad

- 80 grams of cooked chicken.

- 60grams of uncooked quinoa flakes, half a cup.

- 10grams olive oil.

- Lemon zest, thyme and garlic.

- Egg to bind the quinoa flakes.

- Half of a medium tomato, diced.

- 40grams of chickpeas, a quarter cup.

- Half of red capsicum, diced, half a cup.

- Small handful of rocket leaves.

Before getting started on meal prep, you need to know your goals:
- Is it to lose weight?

- Fat loss?

- To build muscle?

- To save cash?

- To get free time during the week?

CHAPTER TWO: Eating Clean

If you want to eat more, shed weight and maintain a healthy lifestyle, then I would advise you not to put this book down just yet. I want you to prep and eat a clean diet for overall wellness. Now that you have learnt something about meal prep, I want to share with you how to eat clean. Far from shedding weight, you will also notice changes in the way you feel, as well as your appearance. This clean diet advocates for eating unprocessed foods, such as veggies, whole grains, lean meats and avoiding artificial foods with preservatives, saturated fat and trans fat. These foods can be prepped and stored as they will not go bad fast; they are natural. All this is accompanied by working out.

When on a clean diet, you will be guided by principles such as:

- Every meal has to contain between 200-300 calories.

- Feed on complex carbs with protein of between 20-21 grams per meal.

- Drink at least eight cups of water on a daily basis.

- Never skip a meal, especially breakfast.

- Take enough healthy fats daily.

Benefits of a clean diet

- Healthier skin -Empty calories from unhealthy foods rob the skin of nutrients that enable it remain strong and glowing. You need to nourish your skin by eating foods with plenty of nutrients and antioxidants.

- Reduced constipation - Processes foods contain no fiber that prevents bloating, constipation and other stomach problems.

- Better mood - Food that are slightly processed have nutrients that support mental wellness. Vitamin B6 found in sunflower seeds and lean poultry support dopamine production, the body feels good chemical.

- Improved flavor - A lot of processed foods have additives that mask natural flavors. Furthermore, other processed foods also have a chemical aftertaste that you can't notice until you get used to a clean diet.

- Boosting brain function - A clean diet nurtures the brain through healthy foods which have vitamins that improve brain functions and have antioxidants that support memory and alertness.

- Higher levels of energy - When you eat foods on a clean diet, you will have much energy while maintaining blood sugar levels.

- Better sleep

- Clean eating also replenishes the digestive system and helps with digestive problems.

- Acne can also be controlled and limited by a clean diet

If you dedicate yourself to the clean diet, you will lose three pounds in seven days. There are foods to avoid when on a clean diet, and they include:

- Over processed foods such as white flour and sugar

- Artificial sweeteners

- Sugary beverages

- Alcohol

- Foods with artificial colorings

- Foods with preservatives

You are advised to shop at farmers' markets or if from a supermarket, select foods with ingredients you are familiar with.

All beginners should know that the leading causes of death such as heart disease, cancer and stroke, are all related to nutrition and the foods that we eat. Your health, weight, levels of energy, mood as well as sleep, is all influenced by diet. It is also important to know that when it comes to food and diet, we can't all agree on a single diet, because our bodies are different, and what works for another may not be fit for the other.

However, when it comes to eating healthy and aiming to lose weight, clean diet is fit for all, because it is about eating real food. The principles of a clean diet are:

- Eating minimally processed foods.

- Eating mostly plants and plant-based foods.

- Eating animal products and animals that mostly feed on plants.

You may be asking yourself how you could identify processed foods. Well, processed foods have the following characteristics:

- They are produced in mass.

- They are consistent from batch to batch.

- Consistent from nation to nation.

- They are made from specialized ingredients.

- All macronutrients are pre-frozen.

- Emulsified.

- They have long shelf-life.

Beginner tips for eating clean

- Prepare your own food – This is the simplest way of controlling what goes into your system. You have the power to control the amount of salt, sugar, flavors and fats that you eat.

- Read the labels – As a beginner, you need to familiarize yourself with the nutrition labels on foods so that you know what the product you are buying contains. Be keen to avoid foods with labels like, "hydrolyzed" or "modified." Look out for labels such as "whole grains". In case the food is high in calories, ensure that the saturated fats as well as the levels of sugar are low, and the calories are from fiber and lean protein.

- Consume whole foods - These are foods that have not been modified or tampered with. Since whole foods are not processed, they have no added sugars, preservatives, fats or salt. Examples of whole foods include fresh fruits and veggies, lean proteins, unsalted nuts and seeds.

- Steer clear of processed foods - They are quite easy to identify because they are mostly packaged in boxes or jars. Processed foods include snack foods such as fries, candy, bottled salad dressing, canned soups as well as flavored nuts among others.

- Eat balanced meals - Make sure that your foods have the right amount of protein, carbs as well as fats because all the three are essential to proper body functions.

Steps to starting a clean diet

- Firstly, you need to know your reason for embarking on a clean diet - Starting on any new diet needs effort and a clean diet is no exception. Therefore, it is important for you as a beginner to know what has inspired you to change. Studies have revealed that the best motivation for inspiring change originates from within, and is rooted in positive thinking. Do not get into a clean diet simply because someone asked you to or because you are feeling guilty about your current dietary habits.

- Determine the amount of time you are willing to commit to the diet - Meaningful changes usually take time. You should know the time you are willing to dedicate to the process; from planning of meals to shopping, food preparation and cooking.

- Audit your current diet- Prepare a food journal and track everything that you eat for at least three days. Tracking your diet will help you make a list of unhealthy as well as nutritious foods.

- Set specific as well as measurable goals - Change your diet gradually

CHAPTER THREE

Recipes

Breakfast

Cake batter chia pudding with coconut whipped cream

This is a gluten-free, vegan and produces two to three servings

Ingredients

- 6 tbsps. chia seeds.

- A cup of unsweetened non-dairy milk, and more for blending.

- 6-8 pitted and well-chopped medjool dates.

- A quarter cup of almond butter.

- A quarter cup of gluten-free rolled oats.

- One and a half tbsps. cacao nibs.

- A tsp. of pure vanilla extract.

- A quarter tsp. almond extract.

Toppings
- A can of full-fat coconut milk (refrigerated overnight).
- 2-4 tsps. pure maple syrup.
- A tsp. pure vanilla extract.

Method of preparation
1. Stir the chia seeds together with the milk and add the dates, almond butter and oats. Cover and keep refrigerated for at least two hours or overnight.

2. Blend the mixture together with cacao nibs, half a tsp. of vanilla and a quarter tsp. of almond. Add a splash of milk and blend until it is creamy and smooth. You may add milk as needed so that the pudding can be as thick as possible.

3. Taste and add half a teaspoon more of vanilla extract if desired, and few drops of almond extract. If you need more sweetness, blend in more chopped dates. Soak the dates for easier blending. Place in the fridge in a sealed container until it is chilled.

4. As you chill, open the can of coconut milk and scrape of the solid white layer. Do not scoop any liquid. Place in a metal bowl and beat with two tsps. of maple syrup and half a teaspoon of vanilla until fluffy. Add more maple and vanilla if needed. Leave it chilled until ready to use and whisk before serving.

5. Serve the pudding with coconut whipped cream on top and sprinkle cacao beans.

Please note that, if you have a blender that is high powered, your dates don't have to be chopped.

Oatmeal with Veggie, Coconut and Maple Sautéed Apples (Gluten-Free and Vegan)

This takes five minutes to prepare, fifteen minutes to cook, so the total time is twenty minutes.

Ingredients
- A cup of rolled oats.
- Three tablespoons veggie seed or more oats.
- A cup of coconut milk.
- A cup of almond milk.
- Pinch of salt.
- Coconut oil or ghee.
- An apple cut into thin slices.
- About a tablespoon of lemon.
- A tablespoon of water.
- Two tablespoons of maple syrup.

- Half a teaspoon of ground cinnamon.

How to prepare

1. Place the oats, veggie, coconut, almond milk and salt in a pot and simmer over medium heat while constantly stirring. Do this until the oats break down, but there is still a little pop left in the veggie. Add more milk as required to keep it creamy and prevent burning.

2. Heat up a little dab of coconut or ghee in a frying pan and add the apples into the pan. Drizzle the lemon juice, water, maple syrup and sprinkle cinnamon. Shake the pan so that you mix the liquids with cinnamon well. Cover the pan and simmer on medium low heat until the apples are soft, but still retain their shape

3. If you want to top it up with flaked coconut, place the coconut in a pan over medium low heat and toast until golden brown, then remove from heat

4. While serving, scoop the oatmeal into bowls and top with soft, sweetened apples and toasted coconut

HEALTHY BANANA BREAD BREAKFAST COOKIES

Nutritional information
- Calories- 60
- Fat- 8g
- Carbs- 12.4g
- Sugar- 2.1g
- Fiber- 1.7g
- Protein- 1.4g

This takes five minutes to prep, ten minutes cook time and fifteen minutes in total for it to be ready.

Ingredients
- Two large smashed bananas
- Two cups of gluten free oats
- Optional - Vanilla extract and beans, chocolate chips, peanut butter chips, butterscotch, dried cranberries, raisins, chopped walnuts, and almonds or cocoa nibs

How to prepare
- Pre-heat the oven to 350°F.

- Blend the oats until they turn to flour.

- Mix the mashed banana and oats in a bowl until smooth. Add half a cup of your desired add in.

- Spray the baking sheet with non-stick spray. Drop dough with large tablespoons and flatten with a rubber spatula. Bake for ten minutes until cookies are set. Remove from the oven and cool on a wire rack.

Lunch

STUFFED ZUCCHINIS WITH TACO FILLING

You can use several variations:
- Ground venison, turkey, chicken or even tofu rather than beef.

- Choose leaner meat.

- If you like spicier zucchini, you may add roasted jalapenos to the taco filling.

Ingredients
- Two tablespoons of butter or olive oil.

- A bell paper that is finely chopped.
- A sweet onion finely chopped.
- Half a teaspoon of salt.
- A quarter teaspoon of pepper.
- A pound of ground meat.

For seasoning
- A tablespoon of cumin.
- Half a teaspoon of paprika.
- Half a teaspoon of garlic powder.
- Half a teaspoon of chili powder.
- Half a teaspoon of salt.
- A quarter teaspoon of pepper.
- A quarter teaspoon of cayenne pepper.
- Mixed cheeses.
- Four or five zucchinis with ends cut off, cut into halves lengthwise and their insides removed.
- Green chopped onions is optional.

How to prepare

1. Pre-heat oven to 400 degrees.

2. Sauté bell pepper, onion, salt and pepper in butter for four minutes over medium heat in a large pan.

3. Mix the seasoning ingredients in a bowl.

4. You then add the ground meat and cook for an additional eight minutes.

5. When the meat is almost done, drain liquid from the pan and add the seasoning ingredients. Cook until the meat is properly cooked.

6. Turn off the heat and mix in one and a half cups of mixed cheeses.

7. Line a rimmed baking sheet with aluminum foil and place zucchini bots on it with the cut side facing up.

8. Sprinkle some olive oil and salt on the inside of each boat for seasoning.

9. Scoop same amounts of meat mixture into the zucchini boats.

10. Cover the boats with a sheet of aluminum foil and cook for a quarter of an hour.

11. Remove the aluminum foil and continue cooking for a further fifteen minutes or until the zucchinis are completely cooked.

12. Top each boat with a tablespoon of cheese and place back in the oven for two more minutes to melt the cheese. Serve with chopped onions.

BERRY, ARUGULA AND QUINOA SALAD WITH LEMON-CHIA SEED DRESSING

Ingredients

Salad

- Three quarter cups of quinoa.
- One and a half cups of water.
- Two cups of arugula.
- A cup of stemmed strawberries cut in half.
- A cup of blueberries.
- A cup of peeled and chopped mango.
- Half a cup of walnuts.
- A tablespoon of chopped fresh mint.

Dressing

1. Two tablespoons of extra virgin oil.
2. Four tablespoons of fresh lemon juice.
3. One and a half teaspoons of chia seeds.

4. A teaspoon of maple syrup or agave.

5. Salt.

6. Pepper.

How to prepare

7. Cook the quinoa. Mix the quinoa and water in a saucepan over medium to high heat. Let it boil and then lower the heat for it to simmer for fifteen minutes or until all the water is absorbed. Remove from the saucepan and leave it covered for five minutes.

8. Prepare the dressing in a small bowl. Mix all the ingredients and set aside.

9. As soon as the quinoa is cooled, prepare the salad. Pour the dressing over the salad and toss gently until well coated.

www.ingramcontent.com/pod-product-compliance
Lightning Source LLC
Chambersburg PA
CBHW071440070526
44578CB00001B/168